Nurses' Aids Series

MICROBIOLOGY FOR NURSES

NAS

NURSES' AIDS SERIES

ANAESTHESIA AND RECOVERY ROOM TECHNIQUES
ANATOMY AND PHYSIOLOGY FOR NURSES
EAR, NOSE AND THROAT NURSING
GASTROENTEROLOGICAL NURSING
GERIATRIC NURSING
MATHEMATICS IN NURSING
MEDICAL NURSING
MICROBIOLOGY FOR NURSES
MULTIPLE CHOICE QUESTIONS, BOOK 1
NEUROMEDICAL AND NEUROSURGICAL NURSING
OBSTETRIC AND GYNAECOLOGICAL NURSING
OPHTHALMIC NURSING
ORTHOPAEDICS FOR NURSES
PAEDIATRIC NURSING
PERSONAL AND COMMUNITY HEALTH
PHARMACOLOGY FOR NURSES
PRACTICAL NURSING
PRACTICAL PROCEDURES FOR NURSES
PSYCHIATRIC NURSING
PSYCHOLOGY FOR NURSES
SOCIOLOGY FOR NURSES
SURGICAL NURSING
THEATRE TECHNIQUE
TROPICAL HYGIENE AND NURSING

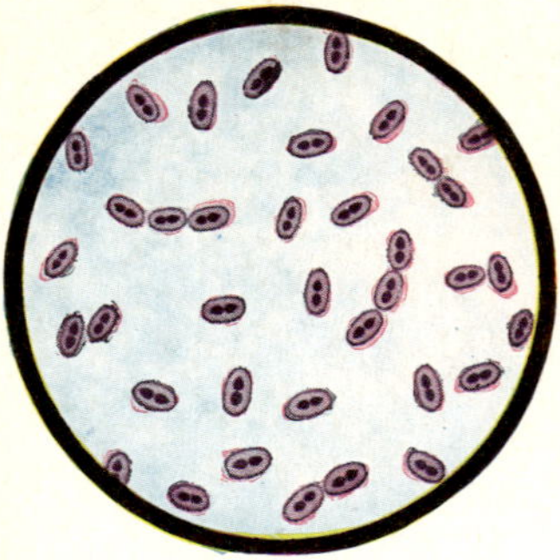

1

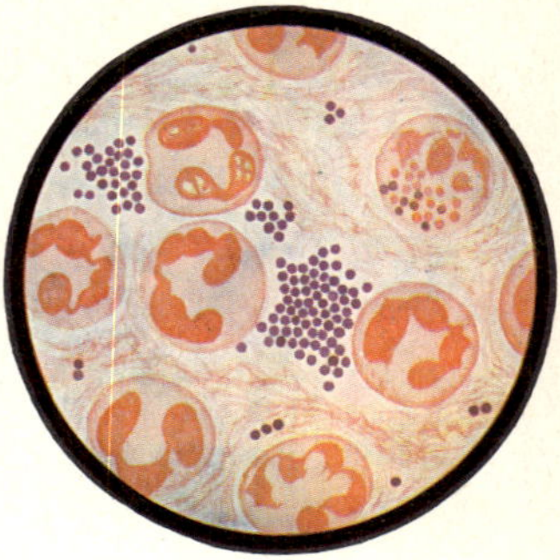

2

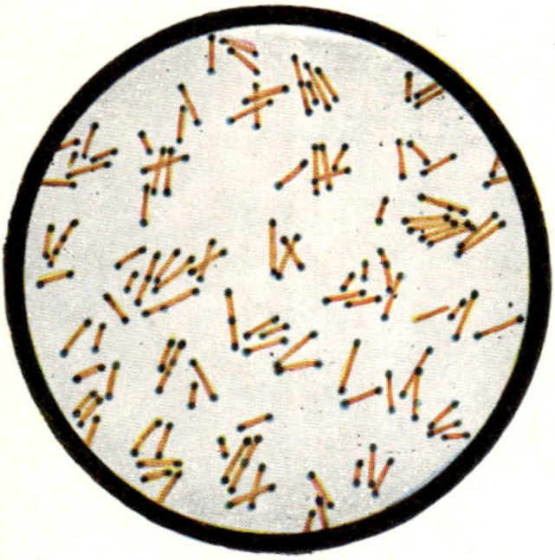

3

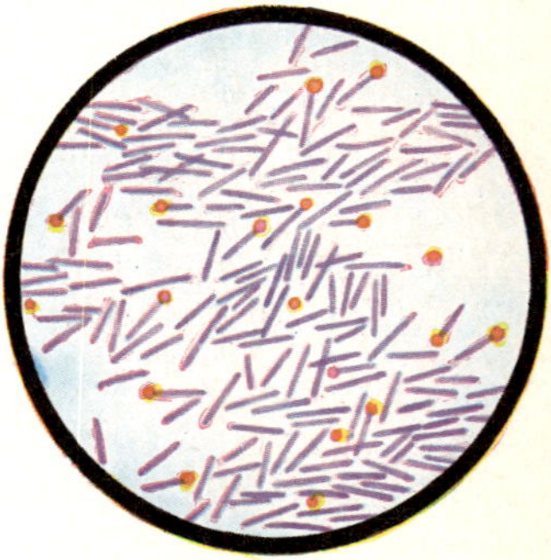

4

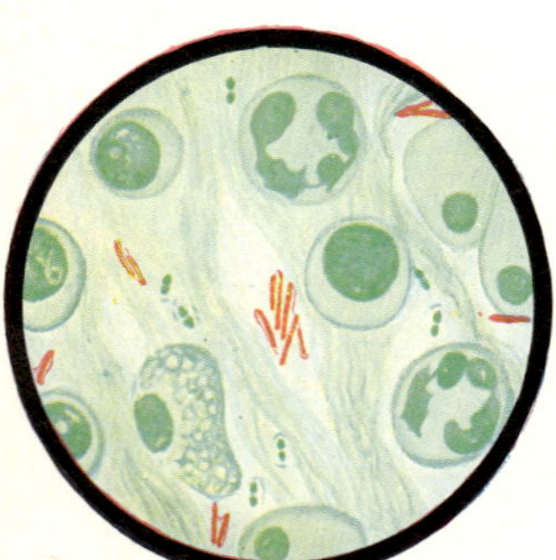

5

1. *Str. pneumoniae* stained to show capsules (see p. 112).
2. Staphylococci in pus (see p. 114).
3. *C. diphtheriae*. Film stained by Neisser's method (see p. 116).
4. *Cl. tetani* stained to show spores (see p. 118).
5. *Myco. tuberculosis* in sputum (see p. 133).

Nurses' Aids Series

Microbiology for Nurses

FIFTH EDITION

Margaret J. Parker, SRN
Nursing Administration (Hospital) Certificate
Nurse Epidemiologist, The Department of Community Medicine, The Middlesex Hospital Medical School, London

FOREWORD BY

R. E. M. Thompson, MB, BS, FRCPATH
Consultant Bacteriologist, The Middlesex Hospital, London
Reader in Bacteriology, The Middlesex Hospital Medical School, London

BAILLIÈRE TINDALL · LONDON

1*

A BAILLIÈRE TINDALL book published by
Cassell & Collier Macmillan Publishers Ltd
35 Red Lion Square, London WC1R 4SG
and at Sydney, Auckland, Toronto, Johannesburg
an affiliate of
Macmillan Publishing Co. Inc.
New York

First published as *Bacteriology for Nurses* 1959
Fourth edition 1972
Reprinted 1972, 1974, 1975, 1976
Fifth edition 1978
Reprinted 1979

ISBN 0 7020 0671 8

ELBS edition: Third edition 1969
Fourth edition 1972
Reprinted 1974, 1976
Fifth edition 1978

ISBN 0 7020 0704 8

Printed in Great Britain by
The Whitefriars Press Ltd., London and Tonbridge

Contents

Foreword

The previous edition, with its special emphasis on infection prevention and control, resulted in a book that proved to be of considerable value to nurses who required some knowledge of microbiology which could be applied easily to the practical ward situation as well as an adequate amount of academic information for examination purposes.

This edition maintains the simple practical approach and I hope that, with the sections altered to increase its ease of understanding, it will prove to be as valuable as its predecessor to all who have to deal with problems related to infection.

April 1977 R. E. M. THOMPSON

**

Preface

I have been encouraged by comments on the fourth edition, made by nurses working in many different situations, to try to include up-to-date information in the new edition without altering the presentation of microbiology as a subject of practical importance to nurses. I hope that this book will be of value to the more advanced student as well as to the majority studying at basic level since all nurses face the same practical problems in maintaining the disciplines of asepsis and in providing a safe environment for patients and staff.

New material has been added to most of the chapters, including a quick reference table of antimicrobial agents, and greater emphasis is placed on the need to observe correct procedures in the collection of specimens for laboratory examination. There is a new chapter on immunity in which the scientific terminology of recent advances in immunology is used, but the immune response and mechanisms are described in an order, and with explanation and examples, which will be readily understood by nurses.

Advice on the text given by three members of the staff of the School of Pathology of The Middlesex Hospital Medical School is particularly appreciated. I should like to thank Dr D. M. S. Dane for further help with the chapter on viruses and Dr Graham Rook for his interest and help in presenting the complex subject of immunity to infection. Dr R. E. M. Thompson, who has kindly written the foreword, is well known as a teacher of microbiology to nurses including many who have studied for the Sister Tutor's Diploma of the University of London at the Royal College of Nursing. I should like to thank him for his teaching and for his interest and guidance in reviewing and preparing this book.

I gratefully acknowledge permission to reproduce illustrations as follows: Figs 1, 2 and 3 from original photographs in the Wellcome Institute of the History of Medicine, by courtesy of the Wellcome Trustees; Fig. 4 from Dr P. N. Cardew; Fig. 9 redrawn from Weir, M. D. *Immunology for Undergraduates,* 1970, by courtesy of Livingstone, Edinburgh; Fig. 30 from Hazen, E. L. and Curtis Read, F. *Laboratory Identification of Pathogenic Fungi Simplified,* 2nd edn, 1960 by courtesy of Charles C. Thomas, Springfield, Illinois.

October 1977 MARGARET J. PARKER

1 Introduction

Microbiology, the study of micro-organisms including bacteria, viruses, rickettsiae, fungi and yeasts, is the study of live cells with very diverse patterns of behaviour and environmental preferences. Some knowledge of their contribution to health (relatively few micro-organisms are disease-producing pathogens), and their dangers and ability to cause disease, is essential to an understanding of the principles by which infection is prevented or controlled. The application of this knowledge to nursing practice is as important a skill as the ability to apply knowledge of physiology to the care of an unconscious patient. Both are a basis for safe nursing care.

Microbiology is a practical subject and not merely one to be mastered for examinations and then dismissed from the mind. The chapters of this book have been designed to bring a just appreciation of the enormous power that minute microscopic and ultra-microscopic organisms have over the lives of men, whether in the field of nursing or in human society as a whole.

The principles of personal and community hygiene are based on an understanding of microbiology. It touches life at every point, from such personal matters as bathing, ventilating a bedroom, and eating habits, to comprehensive public services such as those managed by the local authorities in the supply of water, drainage and building works, or the activities of port sanitary authorities. Microbiological interest stretches from the kitchen where the housewife bottles fruit and makes jam or wine, to the fascinating and detailed preparations of the Arctic explorer whose life will depend upon the preservation of his food supplies, or to the baby whose existence may be threatened by a dirty feeding bottle or teat. Poor hygiene in the home has unpleasant results. Unwashed hands or a dirty, fly-ridden kitchen lead to contamination of food and subsequently to diarrhoea and vomiting in the family; a shared, none-too-clean towel in the bathroom may spread impetigo. Poor hygiene in a hospital has serious, sometimes fatal, results. Because of the lowered resistance of sick patients and the greater concentraton of pathogenic organisms, faulty hygiene is more likely to cause serious outbreaks of infection spreading rapidly amongst the patients, the staff and to the community.

Infection is a hazard to any patient; it prolongs treatment in hospital, with pain or discomfort, loss of working time and income, and worry and inconvenience for the relatives. The economic and social effects on the hospital and the community are considerable, ranging from increased drug and dressing bills, lowered bed occupancy rates and disruption of admission arrangements, to litigation. The emergence of drug-resistant strains of bacteria may be increased by the extensive use of antibiotics in the treatment of the victims.

To nurses more than to most sections of the community is given both the knowledge and the opportunity of practising what has been learnt in this field. This book has been written to further an earnest hope that the practice of nursing will be based in the future on an even more conscientious application of sound microbiological knowledge and principles. Since it has been written for student nurses it has been applied mainly to the hospital field. Nevertheless, the principles it embodies are of the greatest importance in the home, in the community and in every sphere of nursing experience.

2 The History of Microbiology

The history of microbiology is short. Modern ideas on the subject can be said to have started in 1546 when Fracastoro was the first to suggest that infection is composed of minute, insensible particles and is spread by means of them. He noted that the infection was the same for 'he who received as for he who had given' the infection. This was a great advance, recognizing as it did the transmission of disease. Nevertheless, although contagion was generally recognized in some diseases, as in the plague and in syphilis, in others it was still missed.

For centuries all races used the products of bacterial growth and fermentation without realizing the implications of the changes or the processes involved. In fact, the relationship between fermentation and infectious disease was not suspected until two centuries after bacteria were first seen by Antonius van Leeuwenhoek in 1676, using primitive microscopes of his own design and making.

In 1776 Spallanzani first cultivated bacteria in sterilized media, with and without air. He failed, however, to realize the importance of this and either was unaware of Fracastoro's work or failed to relate it to his own.

While this work was being carried on by the scientists, the causation of infectious disease was being investigated empirically by the clinicians of the day. In 1767 John Hunter, investigating the cause of syphilis, experimentally infected himself. Unfortunately he induced a mixed infection of gonorrhoea and syphilis and his results were, because of this, confused. In 1796 Jenner, a pupil of Hunter, introduced vaccination, making use of the practical observation that those who had cowpox were immune or partially immune to smallpox.

In 1847 Semmelweiss, a Viennese obstetrician, realized that puerperal fever was transmitted from one patient to another on the hands of the attendants. He showed conclusively that infection could be greatly reduced by hand-washing and the use of a mild antiseptic (chlorinated lime) on the skin. This discovery is the foundation stone of all modern aseptic techniques in use in hospitals.

A few years later in 1854 Dr John Snow demonstrated that cholera was transmitted through drinking water by showing the geographical relationship of the cases to the Broad Street pump in London and then stopping the outbreak by removing the pump handle.

Improvements in the microscope led to special diseases being associated with certain organisms of characteristic morphology. Davaine in 1850 saw what he called minute 'infusoria' in the blood of sheep dead from anthrax and he was able to transmit the disease by inoculation of greatly diluted blood.

The techniques of modern microbiology were largely initiated and enormously developed by Pasteur, Lister and

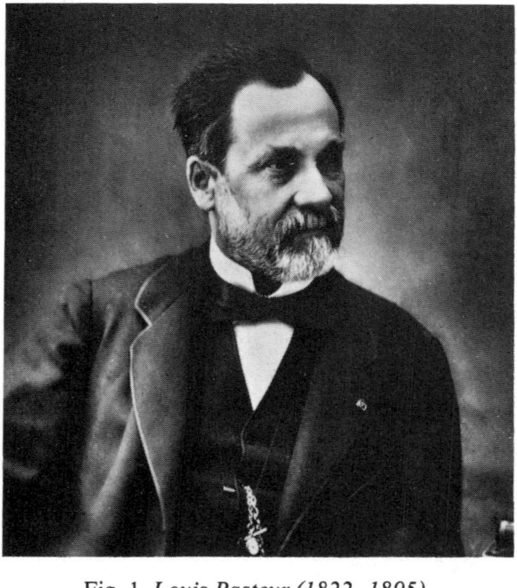

Fig. 1. *Louis Pasteur (1822–1895).*

Koch. Pasteur, a pure chemist, became interested through investigation of industrial fermentation problems. He demonstrated that alcoholic fermentation was brought about by specific bacterial enzymes, and gave a logical explanation for a process which had been carried on for hundreds of years.

Lister followed up Pasteur's work on fermentation and carried out experiments to test the deduction that if fermentation of sugar and starch was due to bacterial action, sepsis and putrefaction of proteins were due to a similar cause. He therefore attempted to prevent bacterial invasion of operation wounds and injuries and the many forms of sepsis which resulted in suppuration, hospital gangrene and septicaemia. He used phenol to destroy germs and prevent them gaining a foothold in wounds. He published the successful results of his work in 1867, though it was many years before many of his sceptical colleagues accepted his teaching. By applying carbolic putty to cases of compound fracture, he was able to save limbs which would previously have been amputated

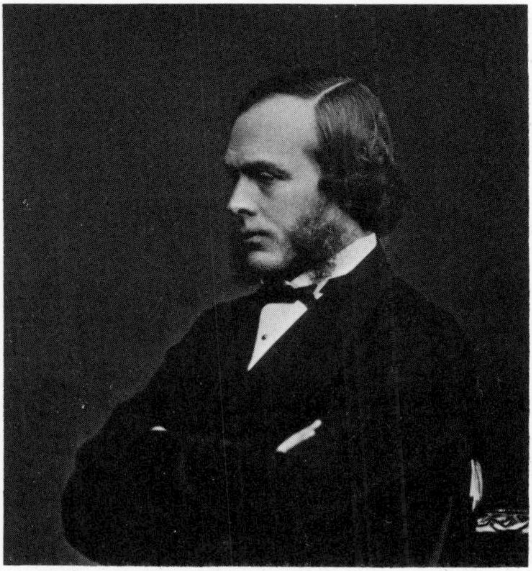

Fig. 2. *Lord Lister (1827–1912).*

because of the risk of a fatal result from gangrene or septicaemia. In the course of his experiments he devised a technique for obtaining pure cultures originating from a single organism, the first man do do so.

While Pasteur was working in France and Lister in England, Koch in Germany was developing the bacteriological techniques which form the basis of modern diagnostic bacteriology. Today it is relatively simple to identify an unknown organism. The necessary tests have been laid down and are simply a matter of applying routine knowledge, but in 1870 Koch had no such rules to help him and new disciplines had to be worked out. Koch isolated the bacillus of anthrax, the first pathogenic organism to be isolated in culture free from other organisms. He devised liquid and solid culture media which include both serum and blood agar and noted that the organisms grew in clusters called colonies which eventually became visible to the naked eye. He saw that these colonies were characteristic and had defined conditions of growth. After this start the causative organisms of numerous other infectious diseases were isolated and their conditions of growth noted in the same way.

In 1881 Klebs and Loeffler isolated the diphtheria bacillus. The discovery of this organism necessitated a reassessment of the preformed theories of bacterial infection. It was discovered that filtrates of growing cultures of this organism, that is to say material in which the organism had been growing but from which it had been removed by means of filtration, were still able to cause death from diphtheria. This led to the discovery of exotoxins, powerful tissue poisons, often enzymes or ferments, which are produced by some organisms during growth and which diffuse into the surrounding tissues to be carried through the body in the blood stream, often to produce injurious effects remote from the site of bacterial growth.

In 1890 von Behring showed that diphtheria could be prevented and cured by the administration of serum from a horse convalescent from diphtheria. This was the

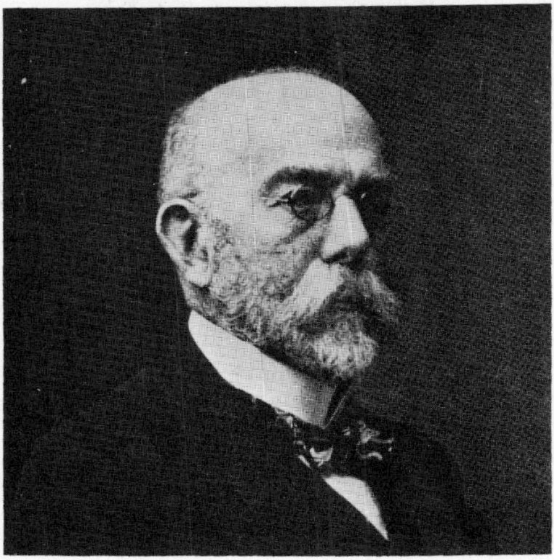

Fig. 3. *Robert Koch (1843–1910).*

discovery of antitoxins. In 1891 Ehrlich standardized diphtheria toxin so that its potency could be assessed and the antitoxin measured against it.

At the beginning of this century Ehrlich was investigating the possibility of finding a 'magic bullet', a chemical sufficiently non-toxic to give to a patient but yet capable of destroying all bacteria in his body. In 1910 he discovered an effective chemotherapeutic agent, the arsenical drug salvarsan 606, able to destroy *Treponema pallidum,* and this was used effectively for many years in the treatment of syphilis.

Following Ehrlich's lead the hunt for chemotherapeutic agents was intensified. In 1935 Domagh found the dye prontosil to be effective against streptococci and this drug and many other members of the same chemical family, the sulphonamides, are still widely used to treat suitable infections. In 1929 Fleming discovered penicillin, which after it had been developed in 1940 by Florey and Chain, proved to be a 'magic bullet' that revolutionized the treatment of infections. The outstanding success of

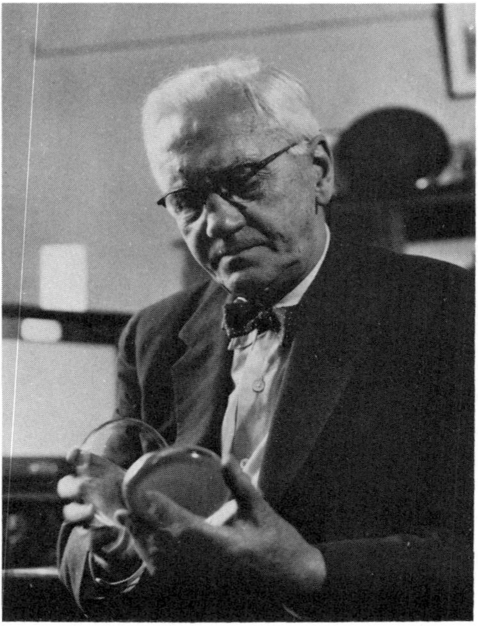

Fig. 4. *Sir Alexander Fleming (1881–1955).*

penicillin stimulated research that has resulted in the discovery of many chemicals and antibiotics effective against bacteria, and doubtless many more will be discovered in the future.

Virology has developed along broadly similar lines to bacteriology, but necessarily more slowly because of the extremely small size of the infective particles and because they can only multiply within living cells. Pasteur, in 1884, did pioneer work on protection against rabies. Loeffler and Trosch showed filterability of foot-and-mouth disease virus through bacteria-retaining filters in 1898. Culture difficulties have been overcome to a considerable extent by the development of tissue culture techniques, and classification of viruses greatly advanced with the development of the electron microscope.

Some outstanding successes in protection have taken place against virus diseases. Notable amongst these are Jenner's vaccination against smallpox, Thailer's yellow fever vaccine, and the Salk (1953) and Sabin (1955) vaccines for poliomyelitis. It is perhaps in the virus field that major advances will occur in the immediate future.

3 The Structure and Function of Micro-organisms

BACTERIA

Bacteria are minute unicellular organisms ranging in size from 0·3 μm to 14 μm in length (1 μm = 0·001 mm). Ten of the smaller organisms could be placed end to end on the diameter of a red cell, and thirty red cells could fit across the diameter of a pin's head; bacteria cannot therefore be seen with the naked eye and the high-power or oil-immersion lens of a microscope is necessary to make out the shape of individual organisms. Each bacterium, however, is a functioning living unit, deriving its food from the surroundings in which it finds itself and using this food to manufacture the complex materials necessary for life and reproduction.

Bacteria vary enormously in the substances which they can utilize as food and there are some bacteria nearly everywhere where active steps have not been taken to remove them – in the soil, in hot springs, in the sea, high in the air, in vegetable matter and on animals and in dust – their type depending upon the available foodstuff and the prevailing physical conditions. Some organisms are particular and require exacting conditions in order to flourish, such as the presence of animals or insects upon which they live; when the existence of the organisms depends upon the presence of these animals or insects, they are said to act as vectors or carriers. The organism causing plague is found in rats; fleas bite the rats, become infected with the bacteria, and convey them to human beings. Ridding an area of rats therefore eliminates plague.

Not all bacteria, however, are harmful; indeed many are essential and a great many are useful. A large group of soil bacteria have the power of using atmospheric nitrogen for their growth; as they grow, reproduce and die, organic nitrogenous material is liberated into the soil enriching it and making it available to plants which do not have this power of 'fixing nitrogen'. Bacteria in the soil elaborate vitamins necessary for animal life, and bacteria in the healthy bowel synthesize vitamins essential to human well-being. Bacteria are used to turn curd or cream into cheese, and the products of yet other bacteria turn grape juice into wine and wine into vinegar. These bacterial reactions are carried out commercially and their products are of benefit to mankind.

The term bacteriology therefore covers the study of a vast number of organisms, by far the greater number of which are not met with in medical work and do not cause disease. Those which are encountered in medical bacteriology have, for generations of organisms and centuries of time, become accustomed to living on organic material or animal tissues, and many have lost the power of using simple inorganic substances as a source of food; they have become to a lesser or greater degree parasitic.

Bacteria are of different shapes,* which can be easily observed when they have been suitably stained and are examined with a high-powered lens on an ordinary microscope. Some varieties are surrounded by a soft jelly-like material, the capsule, which may have a thickness greater than the diameter of the bacteria which it surrounds. Bacteria may be either round, when they are

* The names of different types of bacteria are derived from Greek and Latin words denoting shape or other characteristic, or, in some cases, from the name of the discoverer of the organism. *Bacterium* is derived from Greek, from the diminutive form of the word *baktron,* a rod. The word, however, has been loosely used for all micro-organisms, whatever their shape. *Coccus* is derived from the Greek word *kokkos,* a berry. *Spirochaete* stems from two Greek words: *speiro,* a coil, and *chaite,* flowing hair. *Bacillus* derives from the Latin *baculus,* a rod. Because of the use of the term bacteria for all organisms, bacillus has been widely used for rod-shaped organisms. Although pathologists have returned to the use of bacterium and prefer it to bacillus, the latter term is still much employed in general medicine.

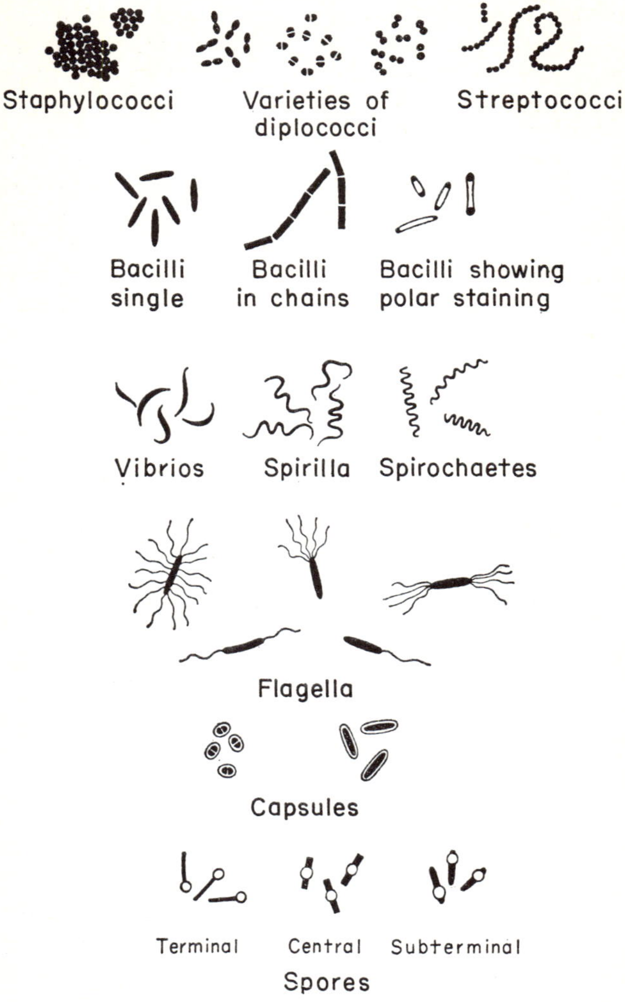

Fig. 5. *Some common bacterial shapes and arrangements.*

said to be coccoid and are often referred to as *cocci,* or rod-shaped, when they may be called *bacilli.* The term *vibrio* is used to describe a micro-organism which is rigid and has a single curve, e.g. the organism that causes cholera. Longer rigid, curved organisms usually with several spirals are termed *spirilla,* while *spirochaetes* are still longer, but flexible, spiral organisms.

The cocci are divided into several groups in accordance with the way in which they are arranged. They may be arranged in clusters, when they are termed *staphylococci,* or in pairs, when the term *diplococci* is applied to them, or in chains, when they are known as *streptococci.*

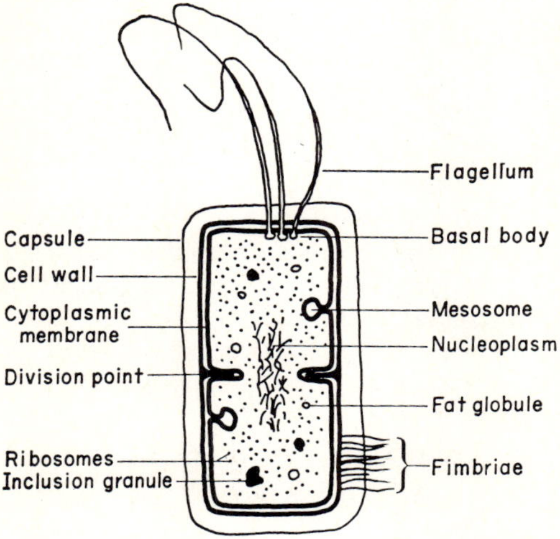

Fig. 6. *The anatomy of a bacterium.*

The detailed anatomy of bacteria is surprisingly complex for what at first glance appears to be a very simple structure. Fig. 6 shows diagrammatically the structures that may be demonstrated in common bacteria with the help of an electron microscope. They consist of a rigid cell wall which preserves the shape of the organism, inside which is a thin flexible cytoplasmic membrane which allows diffusion of liquid to take place between the cell cytoplasm and the environment. The cell contents inside the cytoplasmic membrane are liquid, and contain:

1. The nucleoplasm, nuclear material, or deoxyribonucleic acid (DNA), not bounded by a nuclear membrane as occurs with animal and plant cells.
2. Ribosomes, very numerous tiny granules of ribonucleic acid (RNA) or protein.
3. Mesosomes, granules which sometimes may be formed by invagination of the cytoplasmic membrane.
4. Other inclusion granules and fat globules.
5. Division points, partial septa consisting of cell wall and cell membrane which grow completely across the cell at the time of cell division, thus dividing it into two new cells.

Outside the cell wall may be seen in some species one or more of the following:

1. Flagella, hair-like processes which propel species which possess them by a lashing movement.
2. Capsule, a protective gelatinous layer possibly connected with virulence.
3. Fimbriae, short, stout hair-like processes, not concerned with motility, but possibly with adhesion to host cells.

Bacteria require food and water like other living things. Lack of food and absence of water will cause their death. Some bacteria require oxygen and others will flourish only in its absence. Organisms which require oxygen are termed *aerobes* and those which do not are called *anaerobes*. Bacteria which need oxygen will be found on the surface of wounds and on skin and mucous membranes, for example the organisms which cause sepsis in wounds and produce colds and other respiratory diseases. Bacteria which do not need oxygen and cannot grow in its presence will particularly affect deep wounds such as stab wounds and deep gunshot wounds; they include the bacteria which cause tetanus and gas gangrene. Sometimes these infections may occur in open wounds because there is a mixed infection, and other bacteria present in the wound use up the oxygen available and so produce conditions in which anaerobic organisms can flourish.

Certain groups of organisms, notably those which cause anthrax and the *Clostridium* group responsible for tetanus and gas gangrene, have, in certain circumstances, the power of developing spores, a highly resistant resting phase which can survive for long periods without food or water and resist wide temperature changes and other adverse environmental conditions which would otherwise be fatal. Like the seeds of plants they can grow and mature again when a suitable temperature, food supply and water become available. Spores may be demonstrated easily by ordinary light microscopy.

VIRUSES AND RICKETTSIAE

See Chapter 10 (p. 146).

4 Infection

There are several factors essential to the process of infection:

1. A pathogenic organism, i.e. an organism capable of causing disease.
2. A portal of entry into the host, i.e. a way into the body.
3. Establishment and multiplication within the host, i.e. the way in which the organism spreads within the body, the type of tissue and conditions in which it can grow and multiply. The susceptibility of the host to infection.
4. An exit route from the host.
5. An effective means of transmission, i.e. a way in which the organism can be transferred to another host and thus enabled to survive.

The Organism

Saprophytes are organisms which do not live a parasitic existence but require organic nutriment.

Parasites are organisms living on or in other living organisms which provide the conditions and nutriment necessary for growth and reproduction. They may be:

Commensals (p. 23) and as such harmless in their normal site but capable of causing infection when transferred to an abnormal site, e.g. *Escherichia coli,* a harmless resident of the gut, causes infection in a wound or the bladder.

Pathogens causing diseases. An organism is described as virulent when a very small number produce infection in the host.

Common Portals of Entry

Inhalation through the mouth and nose to the respiratory tract, e.g. the common cold, tuberculosis, diphtheria, influenza.

Ingestion through the mouth to the alimentary tract, e.g. dysentery, brucellosis, poliomyelitis.

Inoculation through the skin or mucous membranes to the deeper tissues. A wider variety of organisms are able to enter the body by this route and to cause conditions ranging from a boil to severe wound infection or virus hepatitis. Healthy intact skin and mucous membranes are natural barriers to infection but when traumatized by accident or by surgical procedure, or devitalized by dietary deficiencies or an inadequate blood supply, they allow the passage of organisms without necessarily appearing to be broken.

Establishment and Reproduction

An organism which has passed a portal of entry stimulates the immune response (p. 26) and may be destroyed or may produce an infectious lesion by further progressive invasion of the tissues or by the production of toxins. Tissue invasion may lead to destruction of tissue cells or mechanically important structures, and in some cases infection spreads through the lymphatic channels to the blood stream (the presence of bacteria in the blood stream = bacteraemia and of virus = viraemia; multiplication of bacteria in the blood stream = septicaemia) and once there, may be carried to other organs such as the kidneys or central nervous system to cause further foci of infection. Many micro-organisms produce toxic enzymes which assist in the process of invasion and tissue destruction.

Some bacteria, while growing, produce a toxin (chemical poison) which interferes with some essential process of the host; for example tetanus toxins affect nerve cells in the spinal cord and diphtheria toxins damage both heart muscle and nervous tissue.

To be an effective pathogenic agent an organism must be able to invade a susceptible host; it can do no harm if it cannot get into the tissues no matter how potentially lethal it may be. It must be able to find a suitable place to multiply before it is killed by the defence mechanisms of the body. *Clostridium welchii* is a normal inhabitant of the faeces and soil and frequently gets into wounds. It comparatively rarely causes disease because it can multiply only under anaerobic conditions, that is where there is no free oxygen. In war wounds and those resulting from road traffic accidents, with much dirt and dead muscle, the conditions become anaerobic, the organisms grow and the disease gas gangrene is produced.

Some organisms, like the haemolytic *Streptococcus,* are relatively unexacting towards the tissues in which they grow, that is to say once they have invaded they can grow and multiply using any tissue in the body as a source of food, and growth will continue unless the organisms are killed by the defences of the body. Others are exacting in their requirements for growth, that is they are more selective and can find the necessary materials only in a particular type of tissue, such as brain tissue in the encephalitis group of viruses or the liver cells in infectious hepatitis. If these exacting organisms do not reach the particular cells in which they can live, they will not produce disease.

Exit and Transmission

Having produced the disease in one host, a pathogen, if it is to continue, must be transmitted to another host or the race will die out. This attribute of communicability is a complex one depending upon many factors, of which only a few can be mentioned here.

Perhaps the most important factor in communicability of pathogenic organisms is the site of the lesion in the infected host or the place of maximum concentration of the organism. If this is in the throat, as for instance with a

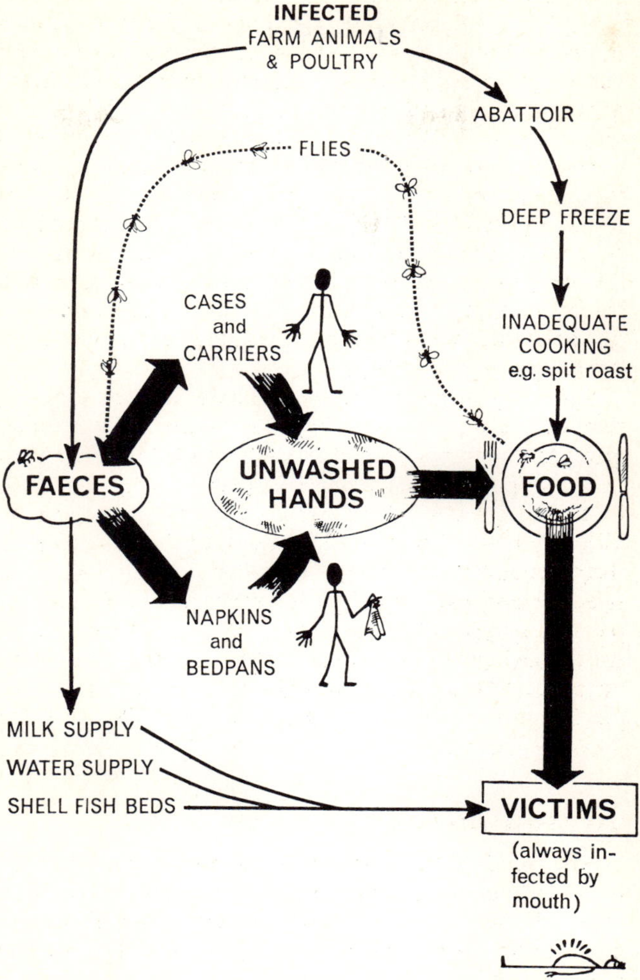

Fig. 7. *Transmission of intestinal infections such as* Salmonella *or* Shigella.

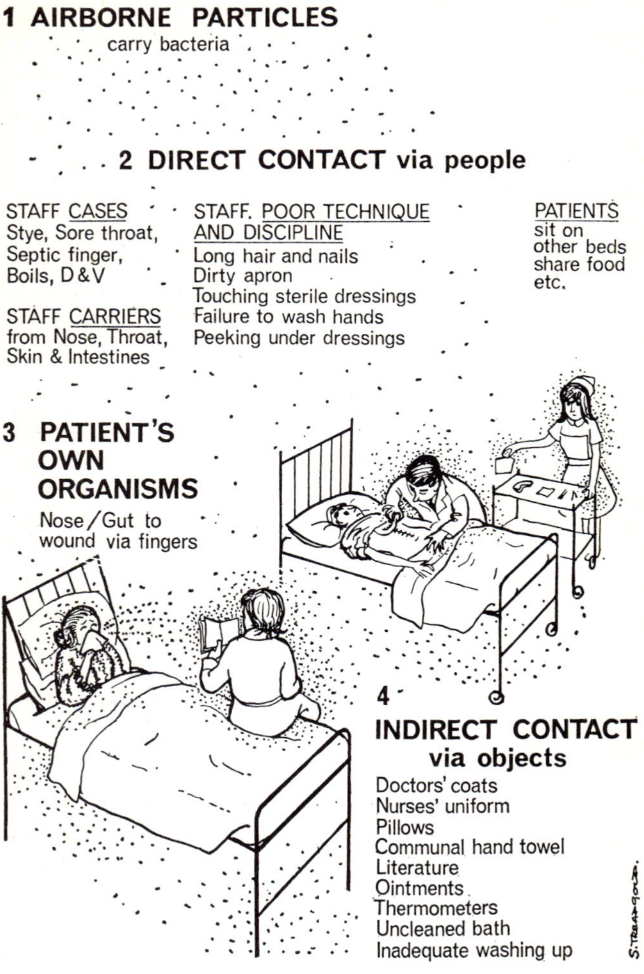

Fig. 8. *Transmission of pathogenic bacteria in a ward.*

haemolytic *Streptococcus* in a case of tonsillitis, this organism will be coughed or breathed into the surrounding air. The force with which it is expelled will determine how far from the infected host the organism will travel.

The same haemolytic *Streptococcus* may have travelled by way of the pharyngotympanic tube into the middle ear, where it has caused inflammation which has spread to the mastoid cells. There is far less likelihood of the organism being transmitted from here because it is bottled up in the bone of the mastoid process, though it will continue to grow and form pus and unless this is released the infection may spread from the mastoid process into the cranial cavity. Again, the same organism may be causing an infection of a finger wound and everything which the infected part touches will have organisms left on it.

If a patient has *Salmonella* food poisoning the organism multiplies in the intestinal tract and is excreted in the faeces from where it can contaminate hands, bed linen, bedpans, or the floor and cleaning equipment. It is important to ensure the safe collection and disposal of the faeces of such patients to prevent the contamination of food or water and further outbreaks of *Salmonella* infection.

Some organisms which cause characteristic diseases in part of the body may be carried in quite another part, where they cause slight or no symptoms but from which they can be easily transmitted. A good example of this is the virus of poliomyelitis. It is a relatively common organism in children and young adults, causing a mild intestinal upset and malaise which is often mistakenly called a 'chill' or 'influenza'. The doctor is often not sent for, so mild is the disease but the organisms are passed in large numbers in the stools. They get on to the hands, thence to food and water. Only occasionally does this organism reach the nerve cells to cause the paralytic cases of classical infantile paralysis but very many cases of this infection could certainly be prevented by thorough washing of the hands before leaving the toilet.

The hepatitis virus is present in the blood and oral

secretions, but also in the faeces of a patient with virus hepatitis though there may be no intestinal symptoms.

Knowledge of the life history of pathogenic organisms makes it possible to take reasonable precautions against infection.

The second important factor in the problem of communicability is the length of time an organism capable of causing disease can live outside the human body. How long can the haemolytic *Steptococcus* live on the sheets when it has been coughed there by the patient with tonsillitis or put there by the septic finger? How long can *Salmonella* organisms live in the stools from the infected patient?

Bacteria vary enormously in the length of time that they can survive in unfavourable conditions and their communicability is profoundly affected by this. The organism of tuberculosis can live for many months protected by mucus in sputum even after this has dried, or in the dust away from sunlight, but the gonococcus, the organism causing gonorrhoea, is killed in half an hour in dry atmospheric air. Gonorrhoea can therefore be transmitted only by direct contact, from patient to patient, while tuberculosis can be caught by inhalation of dust from a room which has previously housed a tuberculosis patient.

If the patient has a disease caused by a pathogenic organism, he is a danger to his fellow men if these organisms can get out and for as long as they are excreted, whether intermittently or continuously. It is not possible to state categorically how long this will be in terms of days or weeks. If the organism is excreted in the urine or faeces, it is these excretions over which special care must be taken during their disposal. A patient with dysentery is excreting the pathogenic organism in his faeces, not by way of his nasal or respiratory secretions, so that no one in contact with him will be protected by wearing a mask. A patient with tuberculosis of the lungs has uninfected stools and no special care need be taken in the disposal of his faeces and urine, but a nurse attending him should wear a mask to prevent the inhalation of coughed-up organisms, and bed linen on which sputum may have fallen is potentially infected and should be safely contained for laundering. In both cases the nurse should wear a gown as the bed linen may be infected, and must wash her hands scrupulously before and after attending to the patient.

Healthy carriers. Patients who have recovered from a disease and who are perfectly well may continue to excrete the pathogenic organism, which causes them no trouble but is a potential source of danger to the community. Such persons are called carriers and are frequently unaware that they are a source of danger and may spread an infectious disease widely, for example a symptom-free nurse or doctor carrying *Streptococcus pyogenes* in the throat; the organisms do not invade but live on the mucous surfaces to be transmitted to another host where conditions may be more suitable for growth and invasion may occur.

It is for this reason that in some occupations involving the handling of food or water, in which pathogenic organisms can be transmitted with ease, the workers are bacteriologically investigated regularly to see if they are carriers of organisms which can be spread in this way, e.g. typhoid excreted in the faeces and spread by unwashed hands.

NORMAL FLORA

The skin and mucous membranes always harbour a variety of micro-organisms because they are in contact with the environment.

Commensal Organisms

Commensal organisms are those which normally live in specific sites of the body without invading the tissues or causing infection. Most are not essential to life but they help to maintain the health and normal function of the body; some intestinal commensals, for example, are known to synthesize vitamin K, others to aid in the absorption of nutrients. They are limited in the body to their own commensal sites and in any other site, even any other commensal site, they may act as pathogens or as transient flora. Thus the commensal organisms of the respiratory tract are different from those of the intestinal tract and both are different from those of the skin:

Examples of Common Commensal Organisms

Upper respiratory tract	*Streptococcus viridans* Diphtheroids *Neisseriae catarrhalis*
Skin	*Staphylococcus albus* Micrococci Diphtheroids
Vagina	Lactobacilli Coliforms *Staphylococcus albus*
Gut	*Bacteroides* sp. *Escherichia coli* *Streptococcus faecalis* *Proteus* sp. Clostridia Lactobacilli Yeasts

Organisms when constantly found in a particular site are also described as the resident flora, e.g. *Staphylococcus albus* lives in the pores of all healthy, undamaged skin without causing infection; they may be called either skin commensals or resident skin flora.

The transient flora consists of non-pathogenic or potentially pathogenic organisms acquired from the environment. They may inhabit a site from seconds to weeks, but do not ordinarily produce infection or disease and do not become permanently established.

If a commensal organism is transferred to another site in the body it may cause infection, e.g. *Escherichia coli* is a normal inhabitant of the gut where it causes neither disease nor infection; if it is transferred to the bladder it will cause a urinary infection.

In certain conditions the surface normally harbouring mixed flora may become damaged or blocked, allowing organisms usually considered to be of low pathogenicity to invade the damaged mucosa and cause disease, e.g. in bronchitic patients whose respiratory tract mucous membrane has been badly damaged by the disease, normal respiratory tract organisms such as *Haemophilus influenzae* are able to invade and cause acute exacerbations of infection.

It is important that hospital staff are aware of commensal organisms and that both they and their patients carry these organisms which may be transferred from their normal sites in the skin, nose, mouth, throat, respiratory tract, vagina and intestine to another vulnerable site where they may cause infection.

5 Immunity

The term immunity in relation to infectious disease derives from the original meaning of the word 'exemption from military service or paying taxes'. It had been recognized from early times that those who had suffered and recovered from infectious disease, e.g. smallpox, measles or diphtheria, were exempt from further attacks of that disease. Such people have developed a *specific immune response* to the infecting organism. The mechanism of this immune response which involves lymphocytes in the lymph nodes and spleen will be discussed in detail later (p. 32). Briefly, in the immune individual, re-exposure to the infection results in rapid recognition and destruction of the organisms before they can cause disease. But this is only true for organisms to which the patient has developed an immune response, as a result of either vaccination or previous infection. There is no such thing as generalized immunity to all infectious diseases. Immunity is specific, that is it indicates the ability of the host to resist one particular invader; for example, the fact that we are told that a patient is immune to diphtheria gives us no information as to his immunity to any other unrelated disease, such as measles or tetanus.

The specific immune response is not the only defence against pathogenic organisms. There are a number of *non-specific mechanisms,* not dependent on previous exposure to the organism, which attempt, not always successfully, to prevent the establishment of infection even in non-immune people. It is when these mechanisms fail that the specific immune response becomes of vital importance. These mechanisms will be discussed in the order corresponding roughly to that in which they would act in an individual exposed to infection for the first time.

Non-specific defence mechanisms

1. Prevention of invasion:
   a. Skin.
   b. Mucous surfaces.
   c. Secretions.
   d. Mechanical arrangement of structures.
2. Non-specific mechanisms following invasion: Inflammation and phagocytosis

Specific immune responses

1. Induction of the immune response.
2. Mechanisms of action of the specific immune response:
   a. B-lymphocytes and antibody production.
   b. T-lymphocytes and cell-mediated immunity.

NON-SPECIFIC DEFENCE MECHANISMS

Prevention of invasion

The body is surrounded by organisms, both pathogenic and non-pathogenic, since they are present on everything we touch and eat and the air we breathe; therefore the skin and mucous surfaces must form the first line of defence.

The skin. The skin has often been said to be impermeable to invasion by pathogenic organisms, but this is only a half-truth. The skin, unlike a sheet of Cellophane, is a complex structure constantly renewing itself and containing hair follicles, sweat and sebaceous glands (Fig. 9). The hair follicles and sweat glands harbour many organisms which it is impossible to remove in spite of the most meticulous treatment, and pathogenic organisms frequently invade from these sites. Axillary abscesses and beard infections are common results of such infection and are difficult to treat. Intact skin does, however, form a barrier against many pathogenic bacteria, and its secretions have antibacterial properties.

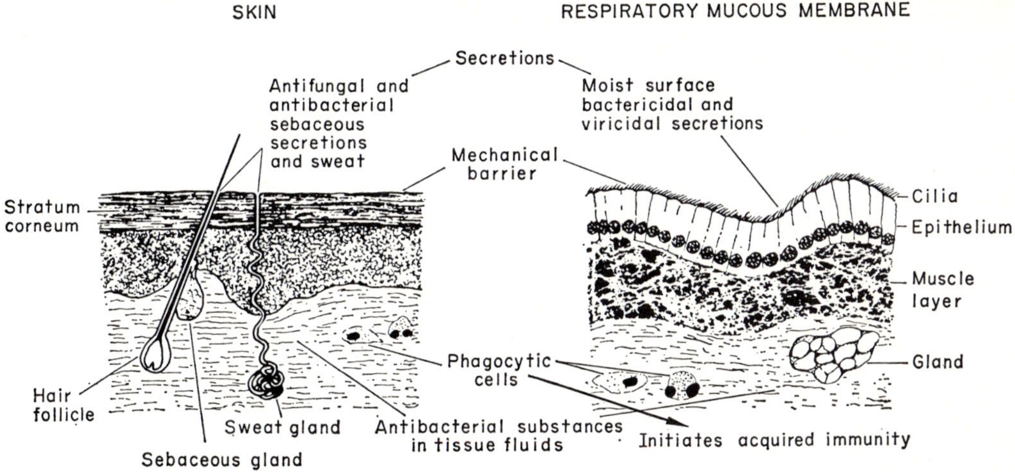

Fig. 9. *The normal defence mechanisms of the skin and respiratory mucous membrane.*

Mucous surfaces. In certain situations where the number of bacteria is high the surfaces are moistened with a mucous secretion to entrap the organisms until they can be removed; the nose, mouth and vagina are good examples of this.

Secretions. All organs in the body which are in contact with the external environment produce secretions. These are most appreciable in places where there is potentially the greatest danger of bacterial invasion. These secretions act in two ways:

1. *By mechanical action.* Secretions of the bronchi entrap organisms and the flow of secretion is moved away from the alveoli by the action of the cilia on the bronchial walls. Tears also wash organisms away from the conjunctivae.

2. *By chemical action of their constituents.* These secretions may be acid, like sweat, adult vaginal secretion and gastric juice, or contain fatty acids, like sweat, or be strongly alkaline, like bile. Abrupt changes from an acid to an alkaline environment are known, for example, to keep the bacterial flora of the alimentary canal in check. Tears and certain other mucosal secretions, for example nasal mucus and saliva, contain an active antibacterial substance, lysozyme.

The mechanical arrangement of structures. As air is inspired it is taken in at high velocity as if by a vacuum cleaner, and this air may contain many pathogenic organisms. The arrangement of the mucus-covered turbinate bones in the nose is such that the air impinges upon them and bacteria stick to the mucous surfaces. The speed of flow of air is considerably reduced, due to the increasing area of the bronchial passages, with the result that by the time the air reaches the alveoli it is travelling very slowly and contains very few organisms. The mucus, swept by the cilia up the air passages into the pharynx, is subsequently swallowed and many of the organisms are killed by the acid in the gastric juice.

The direction of the bronchi may have something to do with the localization of lung infections and the short straight auditory tubes in infants may play a part in the greater frequency of middle ear infections in comparison with infections in adults. The shortness of the urethra in the female compared with that of the male accounts for the ease with which organisms can ascend to the bladder and cause cystitis.

Non-specific Defence Mechanisms Following Invasion

If an organism succeeds in getting through the non-specific barriers above, and so enters the tissues, further non-specific defence mechanisms are activated. These are still not dependent on the specific immune response but, as will be seen later, their efficiency is greatly enhanced by it.

Non-specific inflammation and phagocytosis. Most organisms, once they have entered the tissues, will cause inflammation. The signs of inflammation are heat, redness, swelling and tenderness or pain. These signs are similar whether the tissue irritant is a *Staphylococcus,* a sterile splinter or a chemical irritant.

Capillary dilatation results in an outpouring of fluid, white cells and some red cells from the blood vessels into the tissues. This outpouring of cells and serum is important, since it brings them into contact with the organisms. Serum contains substances which attach non-specifically to the surfaces of many organisms. This can lead, after further interactions with yet another series of serum factors, the *complement system,* to the important consequences shown in Fig. 10.

Once engulfed by phagocytes, the organisms are exposed to toxic molecules and destructive enzymes which usually destroy them, but occasionally the situation is reversed and the organisms kill the phagocytes. Pus is an accumulation of living and dead phagocytes, other blood and tissue cells, cell débris and bacteria.

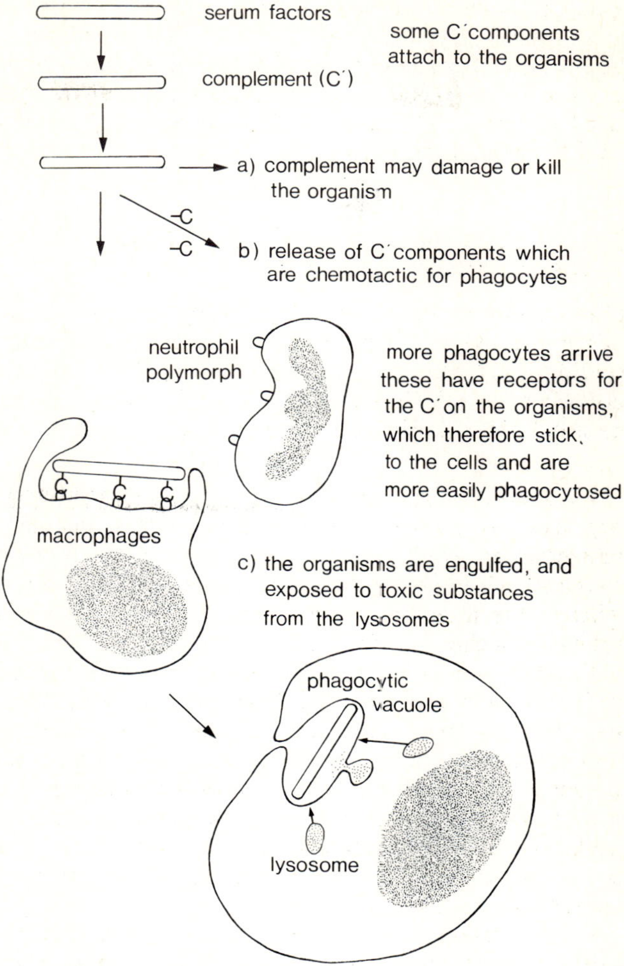

Fig. 10. *Phagocytosis.*

THE SPECIFIC IMMUNE RESPONSE

While the struggle outlined above is going on, the lymphocytes in the lymphoid system are beginning to mount the specific immune response, which then comes to the aid of the non-specific mechanisms.

The Induction of the Immune Response

Stage 1. Every organism is made up of a unique mixture of cell wall components, cytoplasm, enzymes and perhaps toxins. Most of these molecules are unlike anything present in the patient's own tissues and so are recognized as 'foreign'. These are known as *antigens*. Antigens from the infecting organism pass along the lymphatics, free or in macrophages, to the draining lymph nodes.

Stage 2. In the draining lymph node, the antigens come into contact with the surfaces of lymphocytes. Each lymphocyte carries on its surface *receptors* which enable it to recognize one particular type of antigen. When antigen attaches to lymphocytes with receptors of the right specificity the cells begin to proliferate. This proliferation leads to a great increase in the number of lymphocytes able to recognize the antigen in question.

Stage 3. The lymphocytes leave the lymph node via the efferent lymphatics and travel to the site of the infection via the blood stream. Here they assist in the struggle against the infection in a number of ways which are described in the next section.

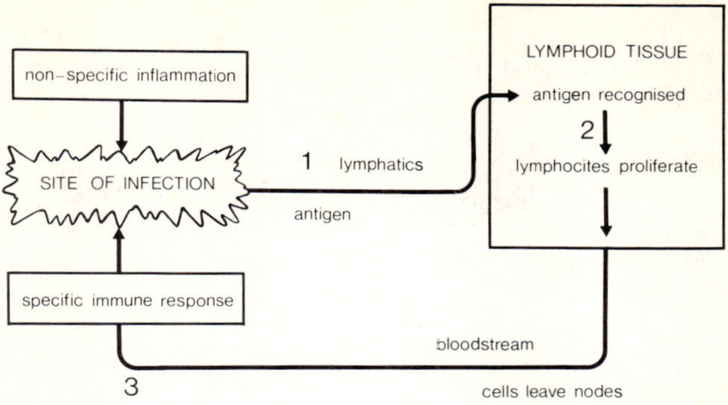

Fig. 11. *Induction of the immune response. Numbers refer to the stages of induction.*

Mechanisms of Action of the Specific Immune Response

B-lymphocytes and antibody production. The lymphocytes discussed above are of two kinds, B-lymphocytes (B-cells) and T-lymphocytes (T-cells).

The B-lymphocytes are the precursors of *antibody-producing cells* (plasma cells). Plasma cells release molecules similar to the antigen-recognizing receptors already described and these molecules, which are referred to as *antibody,* accumulate in the serum and may be present in astonishingly large quantities. Antibodies are subdivided into several classes, each of which has different properties; they are referred to collectively as immunoglobulins. Each antibody molecule has the ability to combine specifically with more antigen of the kind which induced the proliferative lymphocyte response in the draining lymph node. In fact since each antibody molecule may have several antigen-specific combining sites, it may be able to attach to several antigen molecules.

Fig. 12 illustrates the ways in which antibody helps to protect the host.

1. By combining with the active parts of toxins, such as those released in diphtheria or tetanus, antibody can neutralize their effects.

2. Viruses have to attach to cells before they can enter them and cause infection. Antibody can cover the virus and block its ability to do this, e.g. influenza virus.

3. Since each antibody molecule can combine with more than one antigen molecule, antibody can agglutinate antigens or antigen-carrying organisms. Such big clumps of, for instance, small viruses are more easily engulfed by phagocytic cells.

4. Some organisms become coated with complement (p. 30) by means of a direct interaction with various serum factors. Other organisms do not activate complement until antibody molecules have attached to their surfaces. After this has occured, the antigen-bound antibody itself can activate the complement system which leads to attachment of complement to the surface of the organism. Some organisms are lysed by these complement components.

5. Receptors for complement are found on the membranes of phagocytic cells (p. 30). There are also receptors for the free end of antibody molecules, and the 'opsonized' organism thus sticks firmly to macrophages and polymorphs which can then phagocytose the organism very efficiently.

6. Antibody is secreted into the bronchi, the gut and tears and so can reinforce the non-specific barriers such as mucus and cilia (p. 27). Antibody is also secreted in the maternal milk and some subclasses can cross the placenta so that babies are protected for the first few months of life by the mother's antibody. Meanwhile they begin to develop their own immune responses.

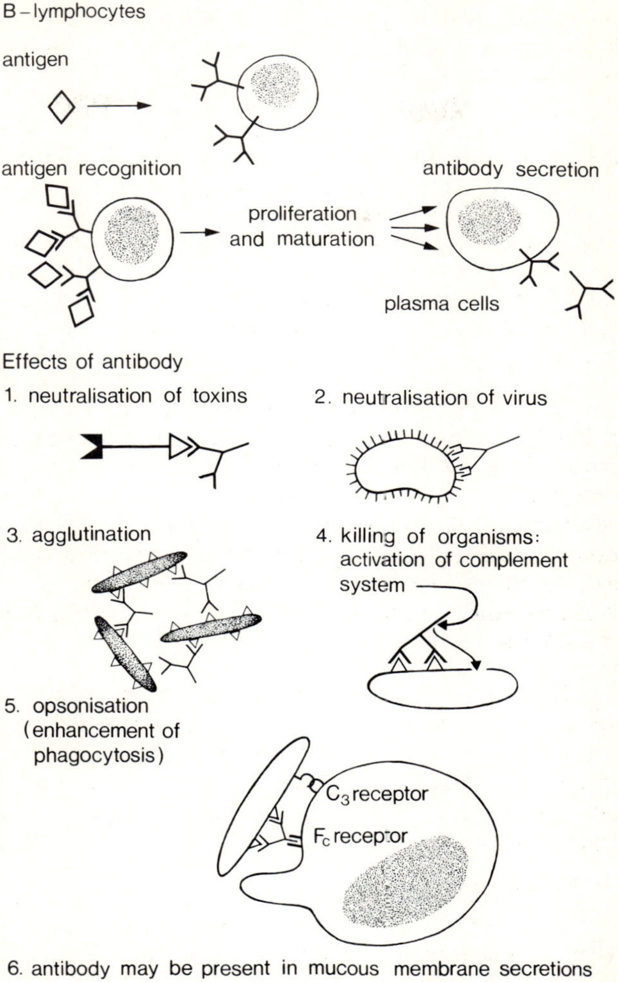

Fig. 12. *B-lymphocyte mechanisms in the specific immune response. Numbers refer to those on p. 34.*

T-lymphocytes and cell-mediated immunity. The T-lymphocytes are so called because they are dependent, particularly in early life, on the presence of the thymus gland. These lymphocytes are absent in the rare children with congenital absence of the thymus and such children have very low resistance to infection, due primarily to loss of *cell-mediated immunity.* As the name suggests, cell-mediated immunity involves the direct interaction of T-lymphocytes with antigen. Unlike the B-cell, where antibody is the antigen-recognizing receptor and the mechanism is known, the T-cell receptor and the way in which it recognizes antigen is not yet fully understood. It is known that T-cell receptors are not antibody.

Two important ways in which T-cell mediated immunity protects the host are illustrated in Fig. 13.

1. When a T-cell encounters the antigen which its receptors recognize, it may release mediators known collectively as lymphokines. The lymphokines make macrophages in the vicinity become activated. This involves a number of complex metabolic changes, the most important of which is an increased ability to destroy micro-organisms. For example tubercle bacilli, even when coated with antibody and complement, appear not to be killed by normal macrophages but activated macrophages can destroy them. This is also the mechanism of defence against leprosy.

2. T-cells and their 'assistants', the activated macrophages, are also able to recognize and damage cells which have become foreign to the host. For instance, virus-infected cells may express viral antigens on to their surface. The cell-mediated response can recognize these antigens and help to localize the infection by attacking such cells and interrupting the virus replication cycle. This mechanism is of particular importance for defence against viruses such as varicella–zoster which can pass directly from cell to cell without being released into the body fluids where they would be exposed to antibody.

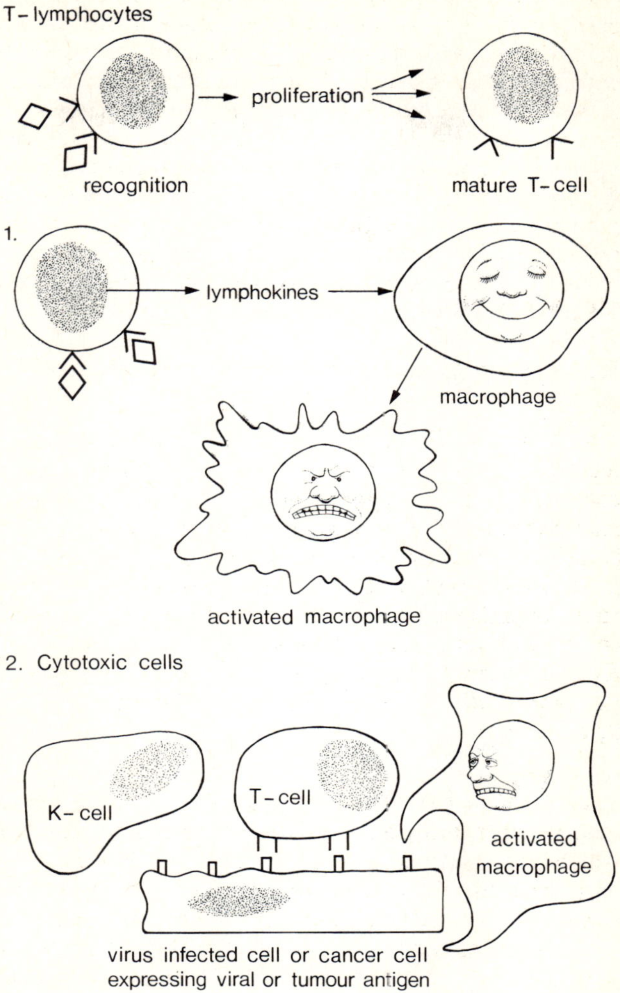

Fig. 13. *T-lymphocyte mechanisms in the specific immune response. Numbers refer to those on p. 36.*

This is why it is common to see an exacerbation of varicella–zoster when T-cell function is compromised, e.g. in patients undergoing cytotoxic therapy.

Similarly, cells which are undergoing mutations or becoming cancerous may alter antigenically and evoke a cell-mediated response. Another recently described cell type which is neither a T-cell nor a B-cell may also be involved in this type of reaction. It is known as a killer or K-cell and its role is still being investigated by immunologists.

SKIN TESTS

If a quantity of antigen too small to cause non-specific inflammation is introduced into the skin of a non-immune individual nothing can be seen at the site of injection.

If the individual has developed a cell-mediated immune response to the antigen in question, T-lymphocytes and macrophages accumulate at the site of injection and cause inflammation, swelling and induration, reaching a peak at 48 or 72 hours. This phenomenon, referred to as delayed hypersensitivity is the basis of the tuberculin test. It can be used to test for cell-mediated responsiveness to many other antigens apart from tuberculin. If the individual has a lot of specific antibody, this will rapidly combine with the antigen, activate complement and cause inflammation which is present within eight hours and then rapidly wanes. Such a reaction is not delayed hypersensitivity; this is why tests are always read at 72 hours since it is the cell-mediated response, rather than the antibody response, which is being checked.

SUMMARY OF THE IMMUNE RESPONSE

The last few pages have described the most important mechanisms which contribute to the immune response. It is essential to realize that during an actual infection all of these mechanisms will play some part, so that an analysis of what is happening at any one time becomes very complicated. This is partly because they are all interrelated. For instance macrophages are important for both antibody responses and cell-mediated responses, and the presence of some antibody and complement is probably essential for the optimal functioning of cell-mediated responses.

If the various mechanisms are understood it is possible to predict the sequence of events in a particular disease. For example, a virus enters by the mouth or respiratory tract and initially infects the mucosa in one of these sites. Physical barriers oppose this, and secreted antibody may prevent it in the immune individual. If the virus succeeds in establishing itself in the cells of the mucosa, it replicates and is released into the blood stream. This is a critical stage. If antibody is present the virus is neutralized, agglutinated and coated with antibody and complement so that it adheres to phagocytes in the blood, liver and spleen via the complement and antibody receptors. It is then rapidly removed and destroyed. In the absence of antibody, the tiny virus particles are not efficiently removed and survive to reach their target organ (the nervous system in poliomyelitis etc.). They then enter cells again, so that antibody is of little help except to mop up any further released virus; the cell-mediated response must take over by recognizing infected cells and limiting local spread. Thus all the mechanisms discussed have occurred in one disease.

VACCINATION AND IMMUNIZATION

Any infectious disease may cause serious complications, even death, and all have some effect on the community in which they occur, for instance school closure or quarantine restrictions or loss of working time. One measure taken to prevent outbreaks and to protect populations against certain diseases is immunization.

Immunization, that is, artificially induced immunity, may be short-term passive immunity or active immunity when the production of specific antibody is stimulated in response to administration of specific antigen but without causing a clinical attack of the disease.

Passive Immunity

Serum from a convalescent person or animal contains specific antibody. This is given:

1. *Therapeutically* to a patient who has already succumbed to the same disease and is not producing sufficient antibody to combat the causative organism or its toxins, e.g. diphtheria antitoxin, antitetanus serum.
2. *Protectively* to a person already at high risk from infection. For instance, susceptible children with conditions such as leukaemia or congenital heart abnormalities are given immunoglobulin (antibody) from a convalescent case, if another child in the ward develops measles. They would be most likely to catch measles, with very serious consequences, if not protected in this way. Similarly, specific hepatitis B immunoglobulin may be given to a member of staff accidentally inoculated with blood from a patient with hepatitis B.

Such immunity is instant but short-term.

Active Immunity

Active immunity is induced by:

1. Suffering from the disease.
2. Inoculation of the organism, or the product of the organism (toxin), responsible for the disease. The organism has to be treated so that it induces the immune response but does not produce the disease.

Vaccines and antitoxins are produced by:

1. Killing the organism, e.g. typhoid.
2. Attenuation of the organism, e.g. BCG, poliomyelitis. Attenuated strains have lost the power to produce invasive infection but induce the same antibody response as fully virulent strains.
3. Modification of exotoxins, e.g. diphtheria, tetanus. In diseases purely due to toxaemia the only antigen capable of inducing the immune response is the exotoxin so that in these disease it is not necessary to inoculate the complete organism. The exotoxin causes the disease and therefore has to be modified before administration. This is usually done by treatment with formaldehyde and the modified toxin is called *toxoid*. Toxoid induces the same immune response as toxin but does not result in symptoms of the disease.

Length of Protection

An attack of a disease or immunization against it does not necessarily confer life-long immunity. The length of protection time varies, but antibody level and therefore resistance to attack is always greatest immediately after recovery from the acute phase of the disease. In streptococcal infections the antibody level falls relatively quickly and further attacks are not uncommon. In other diseases such as measles the antibody level declines equally rapidly but the immune response remains and it is unusual to have more than one attack of the disease. Some infections such as the common cold appear to recur but this is due to the multiplicity of strains of the virus, each antigenically different but each producing comparable symptoms. That is, a series of different colds is due to different antigenic strains not to repeated attacks of the same illness.

Immunization Schedules

The diseases against which routine immunization is advised by the Department of Health and Social Security

(United Kingdom) are diphtheria, pertussis, tetanus, smallpox, poliomyelitis, measles and tuberculosis. Rubella (German measles) immunization should be offered to all girls at the age of 12–13 years who have not had the natural disease because, if they suffer the disease during pregnancy, there is a risk of the infection producing congenital malformations in their babies.

It is unwise to attempt to immunize babies under six months of age because:

1. The immune-response-producing mechanism is not fully developed at this age and therefore antibody production is poor.
2. A high level of maternally transmitted antibody (transplacental and in the milk) may also adversely affect the baby's ability to form antibodies.
3. Severe reactions to the immunizing agents are more likely to occur before this age. On the other hand, it is advisable to immunize children as early as possible because protection is needed most between the ages of one and four years as judged by infectious diseases notification figures.

To reduce the number of visits and the number of injections to a minimum, combined vaccines consisting of mixtures of compatible immunizing agents should be used whenever possible. Fig. 14 provides an acceptable schedule.

Vaccination against smallpox is no longer recommended as a routine procedure in early childhood but it is still recommended for hospital staff.

Routine vaccination against rabies is not usually considered necessary because the long incubation period allows time for prophylactic active immunization after exposure to an infected animal or to the disease.

In order to avoid the risk of travellers introducing infectious diseases, many countries insist upon travellers holding valid immunization certificates on entry. Countries vary a good deal in their requirements, but many require evidence of immunization against some or all of smallpox, cholera and yellow fever. Where these are

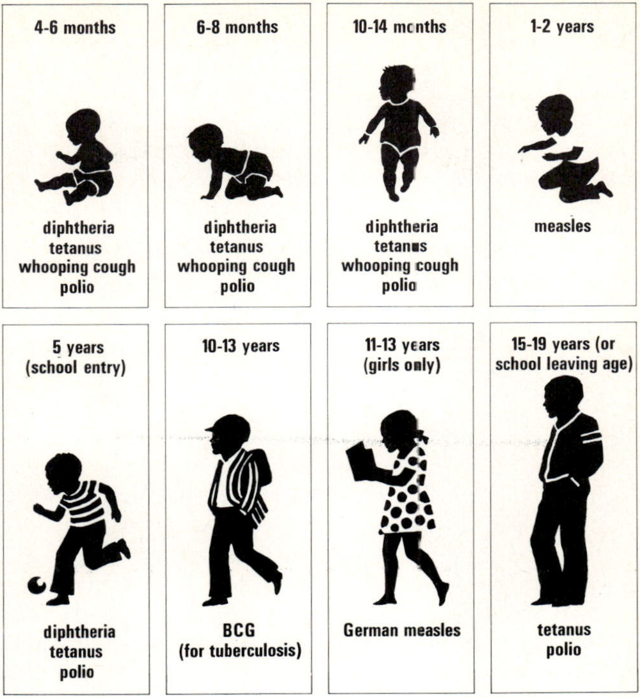

Fig. 14. *The immunization schedule recommended in Great Britain. (By kind permission of* Which?*)*

required, immunizations are valid internationally for three years in the case of smallpox, six months for cholera and ten years for yellow fever.

Detailed information on recommendations and requirements for immunization is given in the following publications:

Department of Health and Social Security (1972) *Immunization against Infectious Diseases*. London: HMSO.

World Health Organization. *Vaccination Requirements for International Travel*. Geneva.

6 Chemotherapy

Treatment of infectious disease by destroying invading micro-organisms within the body was unknown before the pioneer work of Ehrlich at the beginning of this century. In 1904 he succeeded in curing experimental trypanosomiasis (sleeping sickness) by using a dye, trypan red, and in 1910 he showed that the organic arsenical compound salvarsan 606 could cure certain protozoal and spirochaetal infections in man. This latter substance was used successfully in the treatment of syphilis for many years. This was virtually the extent of specific drug therapy against infection for the following 25 years.

The modern era may be said to have begun in 1935 when Domagk reported some success against bacterial diseases due to the β-haemolytic *Streptococcus* with prontosil, a drug of the sulphonamide group. Since 1935 various other drugs belonging to this family have been synthesized to give a wider range of activity against more bacteria, greater potency, less toxicity, and different physicochemical properties, but the action of the whole group is fundamentally the same, depending on the sulphanilamide content. The action of these drugs is bacteriostatic, rather than bactericidal; the organisms are prevented from growing and multiplying and the normal defence mechanisms of the body are enabled to deal with the infection.

In 1940 Woods and Fildes formulated an hypothesis that bacteriostasis occurs by blocking metabolic pathways of the organism. This was based on Woods' observations on the mode of action of sulphonamide. We have seen that bacteria vary enormously in the nutritive material which they can use for building up into bacterial protoplasm and enzymes for breaking down to provide the energy necessary for this synthesis. Some organisms provided with atmospheric nitrogen and carbon can synthesize complex bacterial proteins by an enormous number of chemical changes, each change being catalysed or brought about by a specific enzyme, the process forming a chain of reactions culminating in new bacterial bodies. Loss of an enzyme along this chain of reactions will cause a break in the chain and growth will stop unless the substance is provided in the form of another material, chemically 'nearer' in the chain of the reactions to the bacterial protoplasm, in which case the need for the missing enzyme is eliminated. A substance or chemical group which is necessary for growth of a particular organism is known as an essential metabolite for that organism.

All bacteria which are sensitive to the sulphonamides, and that is a wide range of organisms, require as an essential metabolite *para*-aminobenzoic acid which is a precursor of folic acid. This substance is very similar to sulphanilamide, but sulphanilamide is not biologically active and it cannot take the place of the essential metabolite in the chain of reactions. It is, however, sufficiently similar to react with the enzyme of the bacterial body which uses *para*-aminobenzoic acid. Once the enzyme has reacted with the drug the chain of reactions becomes blocked and growth cannot take place.

In order to produce an effective concentration in the blood, a high dose is given initially, and subsequently reduced to a maintenance level which ensures a high ratio of sulphonamide to *para*-aminobenzoic acid.

If the organism is to survive in a medium flooded with sulphanilamide it must either make its own *para*-aminobenzoic acid from simpler substances or adopt a chain of reactions bypassing the reaction needing *para*-aminobenzoic acid. Both these courses are possible if the bacteria are given sufficient time; they can be trained to do without the essential metabolite and once this resistant strain has been produced, further sulphonamide treatment is useless. It is essential therefore to prevent pathogenic organisms from making these metabolic adjustments, and this is done by flooding the tissues with a sulphonamide. Inadequate therapy and small doses are dangerous, because once a resistant strain has been produced, there is evidence that even in a different host it remains resistant.

Recently a new drug, *trimethoprim,* has been shown to potentiate the action of sulphonamides by blocking the metabolism of folic acid to folinic acid—the next step to that blocked by sulphonamide. Combinations of these drugs (e.g. Co-trimoxazole) are synergistic, that is, they are more effective against sensitive infections than either drug alone or than the simple sum of their separate activities would suggest. Trimethoprim is only prescribed in combination since by itself the drug has low activity and bacteria rapidly develop resistance to it.

Para-aminosalicylic acid (PAS) stands in the same relationship to salicylic acid as the sulphonamides do to *para*-aminobenzoic acid. The growth of virulent tubercle bacilli is stimulated by salicylic acid and inhibited by the closely related substance *para*-aminosalicylic acid.

ANTIBIOTICS

Antibacterial substances which are produced by living cells are known as antibiotics. It has been known for many years that substances produced by various groups of bacteria or moulds will inhibit the growth of other groups of organisms. Many of these substances are also toxic to animal tissues but a few are sufficiently selective in their action against micro-organisms to be used as therapeutic agents. It was not until 1929 that the full importance of these substances began to be recognized.

Penicillin

In 1928, Fleming noticed that colonies of staphylococci were 'dissolved' round a mould of *Penicillin notatum* which was growing by accident on a culture plate. From this mould Florey later extracted the active substance penicillin, the pure form of which is now known as benzylpenicillin. It is supplied as the sodium or potassium salt and is also known as soluble or crystalline penicillin.

Penicillin is very selective in its action and in general it may be said that the Gram-positive cocci and bacilli, the pathogenic Gram-negative cocci and the spirochaetes are sensitive, while the Gram-negative rods and the viruses are penicillin-resistant.

Those organisms which are resistant to penicillin are resistant either because they can grow unharmed in penicillin or because they themselves produce a substance, penicillinase, which destroys penicillin. It is for this reason that treatment by penicillin of a mixed infection due to a sensitive and a resistant organism so often fails. One sees it frequently in varicose ulcers or external ear infections. The primary organism is sensitive, but the lesion becomes secondarily infected with a penicillin-destroying organism.

In all sensitive cultures there are a few organisms which are relatively more resistant than the rest; these arise naturally. In the presence of concentrations of penicillin sufficient to kill the majority, this minority are not killed and they multiply; in this way a resistant strain is established. Since the regular use of penicillin the number of resistant strains of some organisms, particularly staphylococci, has enormously increased; this is why chemotherapy should be reserved for serious infections.

Penicillin has very low toxicity so that very large doses can be given. It is, however, easily inactivated, the newer, purer preparations less so than the older ones. The drug is unstable in solution and its activity rapidly diminishes. Such things as heat, acids, alkalis, alcohol, metals, oxidizing agents, disinfectants and time readily destroy its potency. The dry salt of benzylpenicillin is, however, stable at room temperature. Because of its inactivation by acids, benzylpenicillin is partially destroyed in the stomach, but it may successfully be given by mouth if in sufficiently large doses. For severe infections, however, it must be given by intramuscular injection. It is now considered bad therapy to prescribe small doses of penicillin for local application, e.g. in toothpaste, chewing gum or lozenges which may encourage resistant strains of bacteria and make the patient allergic to the drug.

Penicillin diffuses rapidly through the tissues and an adequate blood level is reached within 15 minutes of an intramuscular injection; the excretion rate through the kidneys is also rapid so that however large a dose of

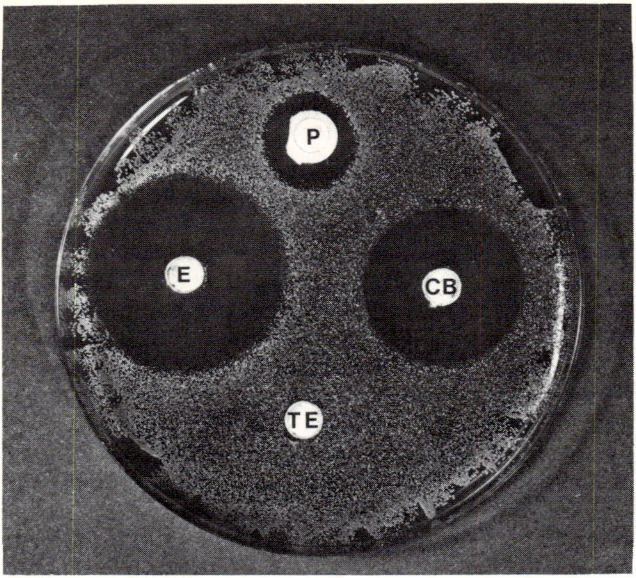

Fig. 15. *Estimation of antibiotic sensitivity. Culture of* Staphylococcus aureus. *Sensitivity indicated by inhibition of growth around discs. P = penicillin; CB = methicillin; TE = tetracycline; and E = erythromycin.*

crystalline penicillin is given the level falls quickly, and after three hours another dose must be given if an adequate level is to be maintained.

Three-hourly injections were wearisome to the patient in hospital and extremely difficult in domicilary cases. Newer preparations (i.e. phenoxymethylpenicillin or penicillin V) are stable in the presence of acid and can thus survive passage through the stomach when given by mouth, and are absorbed from the small gut in an active form. However, none of these is quite as effective as benzylpenicillin, which should always be given for severe sensitive infections.

The basic nucleus of penicillin, 6-aminopenicillanic acid, has been isolated (Batchelor et al. 1959) and it is now possible to produce semi-synthetic modifications. These modifications include:

1. Acid-stable compounds which can be taken by mouth: flucloxacillin, ampicillin, carfecillin.
2. Penicillinase-resistant compounds which will be active in penicillinase-producing staphylococcal infections: methicillin, flucloxacillin.
3. Compounds with broad spectrum activity: ampicillin, amoxycillin.
4. Compounds active against *Pseudomonas aeruginosa*: carbenicillin.

Carfecillin is a variety of penicillin which is acid stable; it is changed to carbenicillin on absorption from the bowel. Carfecillin is specifically prescribed for *Pseudomonas* spp. urinary tract infections but it is not suitable for the treatment of *Pseudomonas* infections in other sites.

The penicillins all act by interfering with bacterial cell wall synthesis.

The Cephalosporins

The *cephalosporins* are a family of antibiotics broadly similar chemically and in their spectrum of activity to the penicillins. The most important indication for their use is hypersensitivity to penicillin, but care must be exercised as such patients may also be sensitive to these drugs.

Aminoglycosides

Since the discovery of penicillin there have been numerous other antibacterial substances produced from soil bacteria, notably the *Streptomyces* group, of which streptomycin was one of the first.

Streptomycin inhibits the growth of nearly all pathogenic organisms with the exception of the spore-bearing organisms, fungi, viruses and rickettsiae; it has therefore the advantage over benzylpenicillin of inhibiting the Gram-negative rods including the coli-typhoid-dysentery group, and also *Mycobacterium tuberculosis*.

Streptomycin is given by intramuscular injection because, although it is more stable than penicillin, it is not absorbed through the gut. Its excretion by the kidneys is not so rapid as penicillin and adequate blood levels can be maintained for 6 to 12 hours after a single injection.

Streptomycin produces serious vestibular disturbances and sometimes deafness after prolonged treatment and less serious toxic symptoms such as nausea and vomiting make it an unpopular drug with patients.

Streptomycin is one of the most active agents in use against tubercle bacilli, and good results have been obtained in tuberculous mengingitis and in acute, generalized or miliary tuberculosis. The main difficulty of streptomycin therapy in tuberculosis and in other diseases is the emergence of streptomycin-resistant strains. For this reason its use is practically restricted to the treatment of tuberculosis and then only in combination with drugs such as *para*-aminosalicylate (PAS) or isoniazid, which prevent the emergence of resistant strains.

Streptomycin is a member of a family of antibiotics, the aminoglycosides, which includes among others the important agents *neomycin, gentamicin, amikacin* and *tobramycin*. Broadly speaking, these agents have the same spectrum of activity as streptomycin, but are more reliably active against infections with Gram-negative bacilli. The toxic effects of these agents are similar to those of streptomycin; neomycin, however, is too toxic for systemic use and is used locally or by mouth in intestinal infections as, like all the members of this family, it is not absorbed from the gut. Gentamicin, tobramycin and amikacin are valuable for the treatment of resistant Gram-negative infections including *Pseudomonas aeruginosa*.

Chloramphenicol

Chloramphenicol, also produced by some strains of streptomyces, is now produced synthetically. It is active against the Gram-positive cocci, Gram-negative bacilli, the organism of relapsing fever, the rickettsiae and some of the larger viruses. The rickettsiae, a group of organisms producing typhus, respond to treatment with chloramphenicol. Other diseases which respond are psittacosis and atypical virus pneumonia.

Chloramphenicol has the advantage of being absorbed

from the gut and for many years has been the drug of choice for the treatment of enteric fever. The main limitation to its use is its liability to cause blood dyscrasias, in particular a fatal aplastic anaemia. For this reason it is restricted in practice to the treatment of certain severe, life-threatening infections.

The Tetracyclines

Important broad-spectrum antibiotics in current use are the tetracyclines (tetracycline, oxytetracycline, chlortetracycline and others). These are all chemical derivatives of the core substance tetracycline and all have similar antibacterial activity and toxic effects.

Chlortetracycline. This antibiotic is produced by another strain of *Streptomyces*. It is well absorbed by mouth and the oral preparations available are stable when kept at room temperature. Injection solutions are less stable and should be freshly prepared. It is active against the Gram-negative bacilli and the Gram-positive and Gram-negative cocci. Certain Gram-negative bacilli such as the *Proteus, Klebsiella* and *Pseudomonas* groups are, however, relatively resistant.

Chlortetracycline causes severe nausea and some diarrhoea in many patients; this can be reduced by giving the drug in milk. *Oxytetracyline* (Terramycin) has a similar range and toxicty to aureomycin.

Broad-spectrum Antimicrobials

Drugs such as chloramphenicol, the tetracyclines and ampicillin have a wide range of antibacterial action, so that their administration inhibits the growth of both pathogens and non-pathogenic organisms which are normally present on the healthy mucous membranes. These non-pathogens play a complex important part in the metabolism of the body. The bacterial flora of the gut and respiratory tract is profoundly altered after giving ampicillin, chloromycetin and chlortetracycline, and this change produces deleterious effects. The normal flora is liable to be replaced by antibiotic-resistant strains of species not normally found in these sites or only normally present in small numbers. For example, the gut flora may become overwhelmed by tetracycline-resistant staphylococci and the patient suffer the acute diarrhoeal disease of staphylococcal enterocolitis as a result, or the fungus *Candida albicans* may run riot in the gut or respiratory tract. In addition there may be vitamin B deficiency associated with the destruction of intestinal bacteria, which produces symptoms of vulval and anal irritation, and there may be vesiculopapular eruptions on the mucous membranes.

Erythromycin, Lincomycin, Clindamycin

These three antibiotics resemble each other in their action against Gram-positive organisms, particularly staphylococci, streptococci and pneumococci. Lincomycin and clindamycin are chemically closely related to each other but not to erythromycin. Despite the similarities there are important differences in the range of action against bacteria. Chief amongst these is that lincomycin and clindamycin are the most active drugs available for the treatment of infections caused by the anaerobic, non-sporing, *Bacteroides* group of organisms. In addition these two related drugs have the valuable property of being, to some degree, concentrated in bone and are therefore suitable for treating bone infections caused by bacteria which are sensitive to them.

Metronidazole

Metronidazole, until recently regarded solely as an antiparasitic agent, widely used in the treatment of *Trichomonas* and certain gut infestations, is now known to be effective in the treatment of anaerobic infections including those due to *Bacteroides* sp.

ANTIFUNGAL AGENTS

Most important antibiotics are produced by fungi, and it is understandable that fungi should be resistant to their effects. There are, however, a few substances that are effective in the treatment of certain human fungus infections. At present the most important of these are nystatin, amphotericin B, flucytosine and griseofulvin.

Nystatin, an almost completely insoluble antibiotic, is effective in the local treatment of moniliasis (infection with *Candida albicans*). It is too insoluble to be injected and it is not absorbed from the intestine, so that its use is restricted to local accessible infection of the mouth, gut and vagina.

Amphotericin B is a soluble, but fairly toxic, antibiotic active against *C. albicans* and a number of other fungi causing systemic infections. On account of its toxicity its use is very largely restricted to the treatment of serious systemic fungal infections.

Flucytosine is absorbed from the intestinal tract and has been used successfully in the treatment of systemic fungal infections due to *C. albicans* and certain other yeast-like fungi.

Griseofulvin is an antibiotic active against the fungi that cause ringworm. It is incorporated and excreted in the skin, thus being of special value in the treatment of fungus infections of difficult skin areas such as the hair and nails.

LIMITATIONS OF ANTIMICROBIAL CHEMOTHERAPY

The administration of almost any drug carries an element of risk to the patient. Inappropriate, inadequate or excessive dosage or an incomplete course of an antibiotic are all likely to have an adverse effect. It is as important for the correct dose to be prescribed and given as it is to select the most appropriate antibiotic to treat an infection.

Too great a concentration of certain antibiotics may have a serious toxic effect such as permanent renal damage or deafness. To reduce this risk blood (serum) antibiotic levels are monitored by laboratory assay at intervals during treatment and the dosage is adjusted as necessary.

An inadequate dose or incomplete course of antibiotic may fail to cure the patient because the amount of the drug absorbed into the tissues is insufficient to combat the invading bacteria; there may then be a relapse, e.g. recurring streptococcal tonsillitis. Another effect of inadequate treatment is that sensitive organisms are destroyed but any survivors are likely to become antibiotic-resistant. This effect is produced, for example, by the indiscriminate application of topical antibiotics to superficial skin lesions, pressure sores and ulcers. Resistant bacteria develop, are transmitted to other patients and cause an outbreak of infection which is very difficult to cure or control. For this reason many hospitals restrict the use of topical antibiotics as a matter of policy and suitable antiseptics are preferred for the treatment of most superficial infections.

More antibiotic substances are rapidly being discovered, and it is becoming apparent that these substances, which are so powerful, have disadvantages as well as advantages. Too little is yet known of the relationship between the metabolism of the normal bacterial flora and the host metabolism, and the administration of one antibiotic may produce an incidental effect on the other organisms on the mucous membranes, with the development of an antibiotic-fast strain of bacteria which may last for many bacterial generations.

To sum up, it is true to say that there are antibiotics now available to deal with the whole pathogenic bacterial kingdom, and the future course of bacterial disease may well depend upon the proper use of the right ones.

Antibiotic treatment cannot replace antiserum treatment in the toxaemias such as tetanus, gas gangrene and diphtheria; the two lines of treatment must go together. The antibiotic inhibits the growth of the organism, but does not neutralize the preformed toxin. The treatment of the virus diseases, however, other than the diseases caused by the large ones, is another matter. Their position, intracellular and out of reach of the tissue fluids, and the fact that their metabolism is so intimately bound up with that of the host metabolism, has so far made many of them immune to available chemotherapeutic agents and antibiotics.

Antimicrobial Chemotherapeutic Agent	*Indications for Use*	*Notes*
PENICILLINS		
Benzyl penicillin (Pen. G)	Gram-positive bacteria; Gram-negative cocci	Parenteral use only
Phenoxymethyl penicillin (Pen. V)	For mild infections as above	Oral only. Absorption variable
Methicillin	Effective against penicillinase-resistant staphylococci	Parenteral use
Flucloxacillin	(Effective against penicillinase-resistant staphylococci)	Parenteral or oral use
Ampicillin	Broad-spectrum activity: coliforms, *Proteus, Str. faecalis, Haemophilus influenzae*	Destroyed by penicillinase-producing staphylococci. May induce a skin rash
Carbenicillin	Many *Ps. aeruginosa* infections	May induce a skin rash
Carfecillin	Specifically *Ps. aeruginosa* urinary tract infections	Oral only. Urinary tract activity only
CEPHALOSPORINS		
Cephaloridine Cephalothin Cephalexin Cephradine	All have broad spectrum activity against Gram-positive and Gram-negative rods and penicillinase-producing staphylococci	Diuretics, especially frusemide, are prescribed with great caution because of the risk of renal failure May be painful injection: cephaloridine or cephalothin Oral, cephalexin; oral/parenteral, cephaloridine
Erythromycin	All are active against staphylococci, streptococci, pneumococci, *Bacteroides*	If erythromycin is the sole antibiotic used *Staph. aureus* may develop resistance
Lincomycin	Bone infections	Lincomycin may cause intestinal upset; give with food
Clindamycin	(Bone infections)	Clindamycin: colitis is a rare toxic effect

Antimicrobial Chemotherapeutic Agent	*Indications for Use*	*Notes*
Fusidic acid	*Staph. aureus* infections	May cause intestinal upset
Tetracycline	Broad-spectrum activity Bacteriostatic	May cause nausea; give in milk Contra-indicated in renal failure and for children (teeth) Toxic effect: diarrhoea
Chloramphenicol	Enteric fever. *H. influenzae* meningitis. Topical eye medications	Toxic effect: aplastic anaemia
Sulphonamides	Wide spectrum of activity	May cause a rash/crystalluria. Always used in combination
Co-trimoxazole (Septrin)	Broad spectrum: streptococci, staphylococci, all Gram-negatives except *Ps. aeruginosa*	Combination of a sulphonamide and trimethoprim. May cause nausea
AMINOGLYCOSIDES		
Streptomycin	Tuberculosis	Toxic effect: 8th cranial nerve damage (vestibular)
Kanamycin		Toxic effect: 8th cranial nerve damage (auditory)
Neomycin	Gut 'sterilization': not absorbed from the bowel	Too toxic for systemic use. Oral/topical
Gentamicin Amikacin Tobramycin	Broad spectrum: serious Gram-negative infections, including *Pseudomonas* spp.	Toxic effect: 8th cranial nerve damage (vestibular). Laboratory assay of serum levels usually ordered to control dosage

Nitrofurantoin Nalidixic acid	Gram-negative urinary tract infections only	May cause nausea
ANTI-TUBERCULOSIS THERAPY		
Streptomycin[1] (see above) Isoniazid[2] *Para*-aminosalicylate[3] (PAS) Rifampicin[4] Ethambutol[5] Thiacetazone[6]	Long term therapy is given in combination, e.g. 1 + 2 + 5/3 for one to two months then 2 + 5/3 + 4 for 18 months or 4 + 2 + 5 all given orally	PAS: large capsule Rifampicin causes red urine, tears, sputum. Given before food for better absorption. May cause a rash or intestinal upset. Antibodies develop after the course so no second course can be given. Thiacetazone successfully used in the developing countries
Metronidazole	*Bacteroides* infections. Anti-parasitic agent	
ANTI-FUNGAL THERAPY		
Nystatin	Moniliasis of mouth, gut, vagina	Insoluble, topical application
Amphotericin B	Serious systemic fungal infections	Very toxic
Flucytosine	Serious systemic fungal infections	Less toxic
Griseofulvin	Ringworm and dermatophytes	Oral use
ANTI-VIRAL THERAPY		
Cytosine arabinoside	Herpesvirus infections	Parenteral
Idoxuridine	Herpesvirus infections	Topical application of limited value
Methisazone	Smallpox contacts	Side effect: nausea. Given only to high-risk, non-immune contacts for very short-term passive immunity

7 Sterilization and Disinfection

Just as organisms vary in the factors and conditions necessary for their growth, so they differ in their response to adverse conditions both physical and chemical. Some are killed easily by short exposure to a relatively low temperature; some, like *Clostridium tetani,* still live after a long exposure to a high temperature. Some organisms, particularly viruses, are relatively susceptible to one type of killing agent, but resistant to another. The sensitivity of an organism to a killing agent is known as the organism's innate susceptibility and it depends upon many factors.

The bacterial kingdom with which the medical microbiologist is concerned can be divided into two parts, this division being based on the Gram stain, as described in Chapter 8. The ability to retain the dye which is shown by the Gram-positive organisms obviously reflects a very different chemical constitution, and the Gram-positive organisms are different in their response to killing agents from the Gram-negative organisms. The Gram-positive group includes a subgroup of organisms which are difficult to kill and which are at the same time highly dangerous to man in certain circumstances. They are the spore-bearing group to which *Cl. tetani, Bacillus anthracis* and *Cl. botulinum* belong.

When assessing a killing agent, the innate susceptibility of the organism it is desired to kill must be considered, and there are other factors which will influence the action of the killing agent:

1. The time necessary for action.
2. The concentration of killing agent.
3. The optimum acidity, or alkalinity for activity of killing agent.

4. The optimum temperature.
5. The numbers of organisms present.
6. The physical state of the material from which it is necessary to remove the bacteria; protein, blood, pus, mucus and dirt act as a protective coat for the bacteria and limit the action of killing agents.
7. Direct contact between all surfaces of the object to be sterilized and the killing agent. Air bubbles in tubing will protect bacteria from steam or chemicals.
8. Antagonistic substances neutralizing the activity of the killing agent.
9. Impurities diluting the agent.
10. Inactivation of the agent by time.

THE CHOICE OF KILLING AGENTS

Choosing a killing agent or bactericide for a particular purpose is a relatively simple matter if the contaminating organism is known. If a child has impetigo due to haemolytic *Streptococcus* the infecting organism must be removed from his toys by some killing agent before the toys are played with by other children. The innate susceptibility of the haemolytic *Streptococcus* is known and the choice of killing agent is wide, the limiting factor being the size and type of material to be disinfected. The particular process is designed to remove the *Streptococcus,* which is a relatively susceptible organism; it will not necessarily remove other more resistant organisms which may be present on the toys, that is to say the toys are not necessarily made sterile or free from all organisms.

The choice of the killing agent to be used against the *Streptococcus* on the skin of the patient, however, is governed by another limiting factor. The agent must be poisonous to the pathogenic organism in concentrations which are not harmful to the patient.

Materials or instruments which are to be introduced into the body, or which touch sites from which pathogenic organisms can get into the body, must be made completely sterile and free from all organisms. Dust contains large numbers of organisms which, being light and small, can be wafted in air currents for long distances. It is not possible to know what organisms are present unless extensive bacteriological tests are done. To be on the safe side, therefore, all materials and instruments to be introduced into the body must be submitted to rigorous sterilizing techniques. The choice of killing agents in these cases is limited to those physical or chemical agents which will kill the most resistant organisms. Sterilization techniques should be checked at frequent intervals (see Appendix I).

DEATH OF MICRO-ORGANISMS

Contact between a sterilizing agent and micro-organisms effects a reduction in the number of organisms; most die, a few survive. If the survivors are exposed to continuous contact with the sterilizing agent virtually all of them will be killed in time. Only a minute percentage of very resistant organisms will survive, perhaps 1 in 10^6 with a marginally acceptable sterilizing method or only 1 in 10^{50} with an efficient method such as autoclaving. The percentage of surviving organisms and the time taken to kill them is dependent on several factors: the number of organisms initially present, the efficiency and reliability of the sterilizing agent and the correct application. A comparatively inefficient agent will take a long time to reduce the number of survivors to an acceptable risk level.

CLEANING

If the number of organisms present affects sterilizing time and efficiency it is clearly of practical importance to reduce the numbers as far as possible before attempting to apply any method of sterilization. It is also essential to remove organic material which will protect bacteria against the action of physical or chemical agents by preventing direct contact.

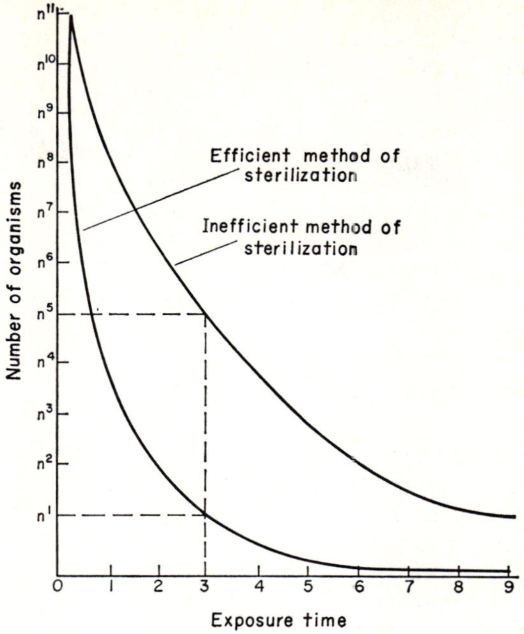

Fig. 16. *With the same exposure time, e.g. 3, an efficient sterilizing method reduces the number of organisms from n^{11} to n^{1}. An inefficient sterilizing method only reduces the number from n^{11} to n^{5}.*

Careful washing of skin, equipment or instruments in plenty of hot water with soap or detergent does not remove all bacteria but it does remove grease and dirt which protect bacteria, and it does effectively reduce the numbers of bacteria. Whenever possible, running water not hot enough to coagulate protein, i.e. $<60°C$, should be used so that bacteria are not simply transferred to the water in the washing bowl. Where there are considerable quantities of equipment to be cleaned, e.g. central sterilizing or central food service departments, automatic jet or deluge washing machines are used to give the most effective wash in a reasonable time.

The development of ultrasonic cleaning equipment for use in hospitals has improved standards of cleaning delicate instruments with ridges and awkward crevices. The source of energy is very high frequency sound waves generated by crystal or magneto-strictive transducers sited in the base of a tank of water to which detergent is added, and in which baskets or racks of instruments are submerged. Cavitation is produced by alternating pressure in the water, the microscopic bubbles of vapour collapsing cause shock waves which dislodge dirt on the submerged instruments. These are subsequently rinsed and dried. The effect of shock waves can be shown by placing a piece of foil on the surface of the water; when the tank is activated pin holes rapidly appear in the foil.

Physical Agents

Heat	Dry	Direct application—Incineration
		Hot air oven
		Infra-red conveyor
	Moist	62°C Pasteurization of milk
		75°C Disinfection of cystoscopes
		80°C Low temperature steam
		100°C Water boiler
		121°C Steam under pressure
Radiation		Ultra-violet light
		Ionizing radiation—Gamma rays
		—Particulate high-energy electrons
Cold		
Drying		
Chemical	Liquids	Halogens
		Heavy metals
		Phenols and cresols
		Chlorinated phenolic (hexachlorophane)
		Chlorhexidine
		Quaternary ammonium compounds
		Alcohols
		Oxidizing agents
		Aldehydes
	Gases	Formaldehyde
		Ethylene oxide
Filtration		

HEAT

Heat resistance of organisms. Different species of micro-organisms vary greatly in their ability to withstand heat. Some such as the gonococcus are very sensitive and will be killed by a few minutes' exposure at 47°C. The majority die after 2–30 min exposure to 50–70°C moist heat. Some, for example *Streptococcus faecalis,* are more resistant and a few with the ability to form spores are very resistant. Since these spore-forming organisms are dangerous to a patient who has sustained an injury or surgery resulting in muscle tissue lacking an adequate oxygen supply, all hospital sterilization procedures aim to kill spore-forming bacteria. Procedures which destroy organisms except the spore formers are described as disinfection or sanitization procedures

Time/temperature relationship. Destruction of micro-organisms by heat is achieved by rapid coagulation of the cell protein with moist heat or by a much slower process of oxidization with dry heat. In either case it is necessary to apply the minimum temperature known to kill, and to maintain this temperature for a definite length of time since the cell wall affords some protection and death is not instantaneous. If the temperature is raised, the exposure time can be decreased. For example a standard time/temperature ratio for moist heat is 121°C for 15 min, if the temperature is raised to 134°C the time required for sterilization is decreased to 3 min (Medical Research Council (1959) Sterilization by steam under increased pressure. *Lancet, i,* 425).

Dry Heat

Dry heat is transferred from source to load by conduction or radiation. High temperatures and comparatively long exposure times are required. These two facts explain why it is not a suitable sterilizing agent for fabrics and dressings which are poor uneven conductors and ruined by excessive heat. It is, however, the method of choice for fine metal cannulae such as lumbar puncture needles and for all glass syringes since these can then be sterilized with a stilette or plunger in position, heating by conduction ensuring sterilization of the inside. Dry heat is also used to sterilize oily pharmaceutical preparations and powders. Sterilizing exposure time is always measured from the point at which the centre of the load attains the required temperature. This will vary according to the size of the load and the type of material being processed, and necessitates careful control and testing of the apparatus (Appendix I).

Direct-application flame. Incineration is the safest method of sterilizing and disposing of infected dressings. Laboratory wire loops used for transferring bacteria and inoculating media are sterilized by heating to redness in a Bunsen burner flame.

Hot air oven. The standard temperature/time ratio is 160°C for 60 min. The total cycle time is considerably longer since it includes the time required for the whole load to attain 160°C prior to exposure time, plus the time required for the load to cool down after sterilization. Hot air ovens used for sterilization must contain a fan to ensure air circulation and thus an even temperature at all levels within the oven.

Infra-red conveyor sterilizer. The standard sterilizing temperature/time ratio is 180°C for 16 min. Metal instruments, needles and glass syringes in containers are placed on a conveyor belt forming the floor of a tunnel, in the roof of which is a series of infra-red heating elements. The speed of the conveyor is regulated to allow heating of the load by radiation and conduction to 180°C and maintenance at this temperature for 16 min.

This apparatus is larger and more difficult to regulate than a hot air oven but in a central department processing large numbers of instruments and syringes has the advantages of continuous processing and speed. Different sizes of containers and contents require adjustments of the conveyor speed or anodization of the larger containers.

Moist Heat

Relatively low temperatures will destroy micro-organisms in the presence of moisture, 121 °C for 15 min exposure to steam under pressure is equivalent in effect to 160 °C for 60 min exposure to dry heat. Temperatures greater than 100 °C are required for reliable sterilization in reasonable time. Pasteurization, boiling, cystoscope 'pasteurization' and tyndallization (a discontinuous steaming process used in the laboratory) do not kill all spore-forming bacteria and are methods of disinfection not sterilization.

Pasteurization. Pasteurization is the method of heat treatment of milk to make it safe for human consumption by removal of pathogenic bacteria such as *Brucella, Streptococcus pyogenes,* or tubercle bacilli which are frequently carried in milk; it is not a method of sterilization, but those organisms which remain after pasteurization are harmless when ingested.

There are two methods of pasteurization in common use in this country. The Holder process entails raising the temperature of the milk to 62 °C, keeping it there for 30 min, then cooling quickly to 13 °C or below. The Flash method keeps the milk at a temperature of not less than 74 °C for 3–5 sec followed by cooling quickly to 13 °C or below. Pasteurization removes the pathogenic bacteria in milk, with the advantage over boiling that it does not alter the taste unpleasantly. In both processes the rapid cooling is important for the keeping properties of the milk as it minimizes multiplication of surviving non-pathogenic bacteria.

Pasteurization of cystoscopes. Many cystoscopes would be damaged by high temperatures and are disinfected, not sterilized, for this reason. The term pasteurization should only be applied to the processing of milk described above but it is colloquially used to describe the total immersion of instruments such as cystoscopes in a water bath at 75 °C for 10 min to destroy non-sporing organisms.

Boiling. Total immersion in boiling water (100°C) for 5 min will kill most pathogenic organisms and is the most reliable method of disinfecting (not sterilizing) instruments and apparatus. It is important to ensure that all items are completely submerged and that no air is trapped within bowls or hollow instruments. No destructive agent, physical or chemical, is effective unless it is in direct contact with all surfaces. Air has the effect of preventing contact and lowering temperature. The required 5 min exposure time is measured from the time when the water actually boils again after the last instruments have been immersed.

Two pairs of Cheatle's or transfer forceps are required for removing instruments or bowls from the boiler after processing. These should be stored in individual containers on a clean shelf adjacent to the boiler, both containers and forceps being cleaned and boiled at least once a day and every time they are contaminated by contact with an unsterile surface. A suitable antiseptic, e.g. Sudol 1–160, sufficient to cover the hinge of the forceps should be added to the container.

Steam under pressure. Steam under pressure as used in autoclaves has physical properties which allow rapid penetration of porous objects and fabrics as well as sterilization of instruments and solid objects. Temperatures greater than the 121°C for 15 min required to kill spores can be readily obtained and this is the commonest and most reliable method of sterilizing dressings, linen, instruments and equipment in hospitals.

PHYSICAL PROPERTIES OF STEAM

Latent heat. The temperature of 1 g of water is raised 1°C by 1 calorie.* 80 calories are required to raise 1 g of water at 20°C to boiling point (100°C). A further 524 calories are required to turn 1 g of water at 100°C to 1 g of steam at the same temperature. These 524 calories are

* It has been internationally agreed that the unit 'joule' should be used to replace the calorie. 1 cal ≈ 4·2 J (joules).

stored in the steam as latent heat. Latent heat is transferred to an object to be sterilized by the steam condensing on the cooler surface as a film of moisture, releasing and transferring the heat instantaneously. This process continues until the object to be sterilized is at the same temperature as the steam; then, sterilization exposure time starts. Steam is able to penetrate porous materials very rapidly provided that it is not impeded by unsuitable wrappings or air trapped within fabrics or hollow instruments.

Air/steam mixture. Air and steam mix by slow diffusion.

When steam is introduced into a vessel such as an autoclave which already contains air, the air being heavier (density 0·12) and cooler than steam (density 0·07) will remain at the bottom of the vessel where the temperature will be significantly lower.

The removal of air from an autoclave during the sterilizing cycle is important for two reasons. Air left in the centre of a pack of linen or in a narrow cannula such as a catheter will prevent the steam from coming into direct contact with the centre towels or the lumen in the centre of the catheter. Failure to contact means failure to sterilize. Secondly, air mixed with steam reduces the temperature of the steam. For example, when a standard pressure of 25 lb/in^2 (1·7 kg/cm^2) of steam is used in an autoclave the relationship of air discharge/temperature/time required for sterilization is shown in the following table:

Air discharge	*Temperature*	*Sterilizing time*
None	115°C	Spores are not killed
1/3	121°C	15 min
2/3	126°C	12 min
Complete	132°C	3 min

Steam pressure. Increasing the pressure of steam in the absence of air increases the temperature. The temperature of steam at 15 lb/in^2 (1·05 kg/cm^2) is 121°C, at 20 lb/in^2 (1·35 kg/cm^2) is 126°C and at 30 lb/in^2 (2·1 kg/cm^2) is 134°C.

Quality of steam. Steam used for sterilizing must have exact characteristics and is described as dry, saturated steam at phase boundary between vapour and water.

Low temperature steam. This is a method of killing all vegetative organisms and most spores present on heat sensitive equipment such as endoscopes or wool blankets. A high vacuum autoclave is modified to admit steam at subatmospheric pressure so that the temperature in the chamber does not rise above 80°C. Exposure times of 30 min to 2 hr are recommended, varying according to the material to be processed. Formaldehyde 38% w/v may be injected into the steam line for increased efficiency.

Autoclaves

Three types of autoclave are widely used in hospitals:

1. Downward displacement for unwrapped instruments.
2. Fluid and laboratory.
3. High vacuum.

They vary from comparatively simple vessels with manually controlled steam inlet and outlet, to highly complex fully automatic machines. Each has a particular function and is used to sterilize a different type of load. All consist basically of a chamber with air-tight doors, constructed to withstand high internal pressures and equipped with a safety valve, controlled steam inlet, chamber drain, thermometer in the outlet drain line, temperature and steam pressure recorders.

Downward displacement autoclave. Steam enters the upper part of the chamber and being lighter, displaces air downwards and out of the drain line. A thermostatic steam trap controls the air and condensate discharge. An autoclave of this type is suitable for unwrapped instrument and surface sterilization. It will not sterilize packs or tubing since air would be trapped within them, preventing steam penetration; nor is it suitable for fabrics

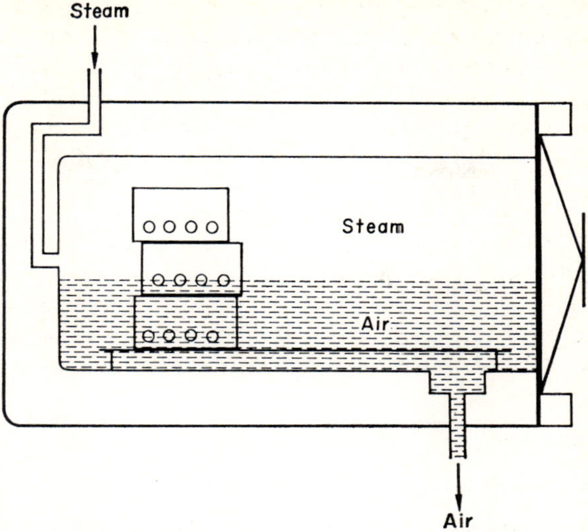

Fig. 17. *Removal of air from an autoclave by downward displacement.*

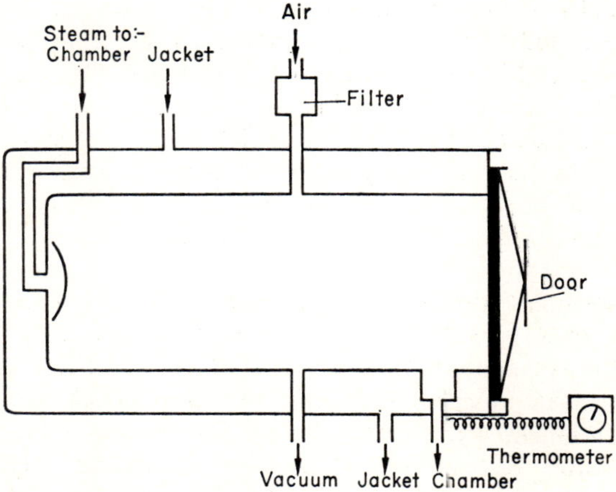

Fig. 18. *Diagrammatic representation of an autoclave.*

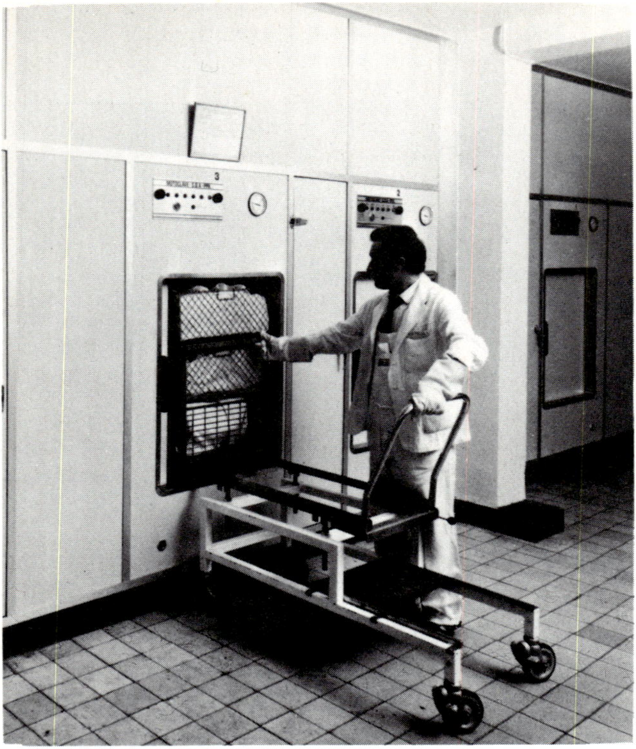

Fig. 19. *A bank of modern high vacuum autoclaves being unloaded in a Central Sterile Supply Department*. (British Sterilizer Co. Ltd.)

and paper which would be wet at the end of the cycle. It is important to load the autoclave carefully to facilitate air displacement and free steam circulation.

Autoclaves for fluids and laboratory use. These autoclaves operate on the same principle as the displacement type but usually can be operated at a variety of steam pressures thus allowing a wider range of temperature settings. They often have a slow exhaust cycle to prevent fluids from 'boiling' over or bottles from exploding. Some models have a post-sterilization water cooling cycle which shortens the total time by cooling the outside of the sterilized bottles and allows the operator to open the autoclave door at the end of the cycle without risk of cooler room air in contact with extremely hot bottles causing explosion and injury. They should be fitted with an inner safety door for the same reason.

Bottles of fluids prepared for sterilization should be three quarters filled, and capped. Sterilization exposure time depends on the size of the container. For example at 121°C a 500 ml bottle requires 24 min while a 2000 ml bottle requires 40 min exposure.

High vacuum autoclaves. These are very complex, automatically operated, jacketed autoclaves designed for efficient, fast sterilization of air-trapping loads such as packs of fabrics, dressings and instruments, limited lengths of tubing and hollow equipment. The complexity of the machines and the critical importance of air displacement from the load make regular skilled maintenance and testing essential to safe sterilizing practice (Appendix I).

High vacuum autoclave cycle. The autoclave is loaded and the automatic cycle, which in modern machines includes door closure, is started. Air contained within the chamber, within the packs and their contents, is pumped out through the outlet drain, i.e. a vacuum is drawn to reduce the pressure from 760 mmHg (100 kPa) (atmospheric) to less than 20 mmHg (2·5 kPa) in the chamber. A minute amount of air (< 3%) remains. Air is much more easily and quickly displaced from the space surrounding the load than from the centre of the packs and their contents. It follows that if the autoclave is loaded with only one or two small packs, there is a danger that the residual air will be concentrated in the centre of the packs where it will prevent steam penetration and therefore sterilization. To increase efficiency and to safeguard against this 'small load phenomenon' a steam pulsing phase has been added to most high vacuum autoclave cycles. At the beginning of the sterilizing phase, steam under pressure is pulsed into, and withdrawn from, the chamber in a series of six rapid bursts to ensure movement and diffusion of any remaining air. Because of the vacuum steam is immediately able to penetrate to the centre of the packs and equipment. Sterilization exposure time (p. 63) is measured from the point at which the load attains the same temperature as the steam, usually 134 °C for 3 min. A second or post-sterilizing vacuum is drawn to remove the steam from the load. Filtered sterile air is then allowed into the chamber to replace the vacuum, maintaining the sterility of the load.

A porous load autoclave is surrounded by a steam insulating jacket which is not connected to the chamber. Its function is to prevent heat loss during the sterilizing phase and to assist in the rapid drying of the load which occurs during the post-sterilizing vacuum, and vacuum breaking phases. The steam supply to the jacket is not normally turned off, the jacket is therefore constantly at sterilizing temperature. Excessive drying of the load, damage to fabrics, and sterilizing failures due to the superheated steam will occur if the load is held in the autoclave for any length of time prior to starting the cycle.

RADIATION

Ultra-violet Light

Prolonged exposure to fresh air and sunlight is perhaps the oldest and most pleasant anti-infection measure. Ultra-violet rays reduce the number of air-borne bacteria but the practical value of an ultra-violet light installation as a means of killing bacteria in a hospital is minimal and its efficiency limited by disadvantageous physical properties.

1. Light travels in straight lines and does not penetrate. Only the surface of an object in direct line with the ultra-violet source is irradiated, any bacteria in 'the shadows' are totally unaffected.

2. Direct exposure to ultra-violet light causes conjunctival damage, so that either dark glasses must be worn or the light source screened.

3. Bacterial kill is not instantaneous. Neither human beings nor air passing at normal speed through a doorway with an overhead source will receive adequate exposure.

Ionizing Radiation

The scientific exploration and development of the peaceful uses of atomic energy is a twentieth century achievement which has made considerable contributions to the advancement of medical technology. In the field of sterilization, particularly in the United Kingdom, a very reliable means of sterilizing thermolabile (heat-sensitive) materials has become commercially available at a reasonable cost. The size of the plant, the cost of the source, and the statutory safeguards required in the handling of radioactive materials determine that the method is nationally and commercially, rather than hospital centred.

Sources. Two sources of ionizing radiation are now used:

1. Gamma rays from the radioisotope cobalt 60.
2. Particulate high-energy electrons from a linear accelerator.

Gamma rays have the greater power of penetration so that while standard medical packs for gamma irradiation are up to 30 cm thick, those for electron beam processing are usually single, small items. Penetration in both cases is dependent on the density of the material being processed; standard packs allow for mixed contents.

The plants are fully automatic to avoid exposing operators to ionizing radiation. Conveyor belts carry standard sized packs, at standard speed, past the source so that each pack receives a measured dose. It is usual for packs to be automatically turned and irrdiated from more than one side in such a plant.

Dose. The International Atomic Energy Agency of the United Nations Working Party recommended code of practice for radiation sterilization 1967, covers many aspects of packaging and plant control including the dose requirement. In the United Kingdom and several other countries a radiation sterilization dose of 2·5 Mrad has been in use for medical disposable products for over ten years. At this dosage it is important that articles to be sterilized are, as far as possible, free from living virus particles. This is because the dosage of radiation required to kill micro-organisms is inversely proportional to the particle size, i.e. a larger dose of radiation is required to kill a small virus particle than to kill a large bacterial particle.

A rad is a unit of measurement of energy absorbed from radiation by the matter through which it passes. 1 rad involves the liberation of 100 ergs of energy into each gram. In practical terms this means that the rise in temperature during sterilization is only a few degrees C. 1 Mrad = 1 million rads.

Suitable materials. Ionizing radiation never induces radioactivity in the materials being processed but it does induce chemical changes in some materials making them temporarily or permanently unstable and therefore unsuited to the process. Teflon (PTFE) is an example of permanent damage and sugar, which turns pink but reverts, is an example of temporary instability.

One of the great benefits to the medical field is the safe sterilization of the increasing numbers of disposable plastic items such as syringes and catheters which will not withstand heat sterilization, and sharps such as hypodermic needles and scalpel blades. These can now be packed before sterilization in individual sealed aluminium foil or plastic packs contained in an outer carbon carton ready for dispatch, avoiding any handling and possible recontamination after sterilization.

COLD

Freezing as a method of killing micro-organisms is not satisfactory for ordinary use because the survival rate of organisms in low temperatures varies considerably. Refrigeration is, however, an excellent method for preserving food, sera, etc., when the temperature is kept at about 4°C. Organisms are not killed by this method but they do not multiply. Perishable goods should be placed in the refrigerator immediately. If they are allowed to stay in a warm atmosphere for several hours organisms present in them will have a chance of multiplying and refrigeration after this time will be useless. Preformed toxins are not destroyed by refrigeration and no amount of cooling after they have been formed will make the food safe to eat.

DRYING

Many organisms are killed by drying and this factor limits the natural spread of many diseases. Spores, however, can withstand remaining dry for many months or even years and, as a practical method of killing bacteria, drying is unsatisfactory.

CHEMICAL AGENTS

There are a bewildering number of chemical preparations on the market. Very few of them are reliable *sterilizing agents* (i.e. remove or destroy all micro-organisms) in the strengths and under the circumstances in which they are used in the home or in hospital. The term *disinfectant* usually describes those which are capable of removing or killing micro-organisms on inanimate objects not usually including bacterial spores. An *antiseptic* inhibits micro-organisms (i.e. prevents growth and multiplication). The term antiseptic is used of weaker and less toxic solutions which inhibit, and may kill. It is commonly used to describe applications to living tissue. *Germicide* is a newer word meaning a chemical capable of killing micro-organisms.

The suffix *-cide* indicates that an agent kills. Bactericides kill bacteria. Fungicides kill fungi.

The suffix *-stat* indicates that an agent prevents or inhibits growth.

No single preparation fulfills all requirements and all are less reliable than heat or radiation as sterilizing agents.

Too often the choice of chemical agent is a matter of whim or fashion which results in unjustifiable expense and inefficient practice. It is helpful if a committee such as a hospital control of infection committee which includes a pharmacist is responsible for advising on the selection and use of disinfectants, germicides and antiseptics. The aim of the committee should be to select efficient agents, to define the dilutions and exposure times appropriate to specific uses, and to limit the number of agents purchased.

In making an assessment consideration should be given to several important factors:

1. The need: (*a*) Decontamination of inanimate objects such as floors, furniture, kitchen equipment, infected linen, medical and nursing equipment. (*b*) Decontamination of living tissue such as skin, wounds, eyes, body cavities.
2. Any known local conditions or problems, e.g. a high incidence of staphylococcal infection, a tuberculosis unit. Some organisms are very resistant to the action of chemical agents, e.g. *Pseudomonas aeruginosa*.
3. The efficiency of the agents, basing judgements on in-use tests (Kelsey & Maurer 1974), i.e. the performance in clean and dirty working situations (see Appendix I).
4. Safety for both patients and staff. Preferably chemicals which are neither irritant, toxic, nor corrosive.
5. The degree of hardness of the local water to be used for dilution purposes. This may affect the efficiency of the agent.
6. Stability during storage and in use.
7. Time taken to act.
8. Any other problems produced by use, e.g. staining

of bed and personal linen, corrosion of metal, sensitization.

9. Cost.

Guide lines for use should include reminders:

1. Never use chemicals if more reliable methods are available.
2. Cleaning is the first and most important step in chemical disinfection.
3. Total surface contact is essential.
4. Recommended strengths for specific purposes, i.e. clean and dirty situations.
5. No agent acts instantaneously. Note the recommended exposure time.
6. Equipment has to be rinsed after immersion in a chemical. It is very easy to recontaminate it at this stage unless sterile water, dishes and forceps are used.
7. Antiseptics and ointments may themselves become contaminated by incorrect use, e.g. by placing a hand or swab on the top of a bottle or by dipping fingers into containers of ointment or cream. They vary in antimicrobial activity and are not effective against every type of organism which may be picked up and transferred by hands.

Some Common Preparations—Liquids

The Halogens. *Iodine* 2·5% in 70% alcohol is perhaps the most effective skin germicide but it is an irritant and may cause a severe reaction in a sensitive subject and has the further disadvantage of staining. The *iodophors,* e.g. povidone-iodine (Betadine, Wescodyne), are combinations of iodine and non-ionic detergents. They have the good properties of iodine but are non-staining, much less toxic, and less irritant. The solutions contain a colour indicator which fades as the germicidal activity diminishes.

Chlorine compounds such as chlorinated lime, chloramines, and hypochlorites, are capable of liberating active chlorine. *Chlorinated lime* or domestic bleach is used for disinfecting drinking water, swimming baths, drains, etc. Since chlorine compounds are relatively easily inhibited by organic matter it is important to keep drain traps and overflows clean in addition to using the disinfectant. *Eusol* is a chlorinated lime and boric acid compound used for wound dressings and packs but is usually considered to be too irritant for irrigation purposes. *Dakin's solution* (surgical chlorinated soda solution BPC) and ESH (electrolytic sodium hypochlorite) are used for wound irrigation and dressings. Milton 1% (sodium hypochlorite) is also commonly used to disinfect baby bottles and for kitchen hygiene. Hypochlorites are effective against most viruses.

Heavy metals. Silver nitrate 1% is currently widely used in the treatment of burns. A practical disadvantage is the indelible black staining of bed and personal linen.

Phenol and cresol compounds. These are coal tar derivatives which have been in use in hospitals for over a hundred years. Phenol (carbolic acid) used by Lord Lister to destroy bacteria in wounds and to prevent their access to wounds (*Lancet* 1867) was more recently used as the standard disinfectant against which the efficiency and activity of others was measured in the Rideal-Walker test (1903). It is not now used for wounds since it is toxic and irritant and may cause local tissue damage and remote kidney damage.

Modern phenolic compounds, e.g. *Hycolin* 1%, are more efficient than phenol and have fewer disadvantages.

Lysol, Sudol, Jeye's fluid and *Cyllin* are saponified or emulsified solutions of cresol compounds. They are effective, relatively cheap and suitable for floor and surface disinfection and for decontamination of infected linen. The soap content enhances the action but will precipitate if the solution is diluted with hard water. In strong solution these agents, especially lysol, will damage the skin and eyes and therefore require careful handling.

Chlorinated Phenolic. *Hexachlorophane* is a chlorinated phenolic bacteriostatic agent which was widely used combined with a compatible soap for skin cleansing, in particular hand-washing, in operating theatres and clinical areas. It is cumulative in action and is therefore most effective when used consistently and frequently. Hexachlorophane is very poorly soluble in water and is precipitated on to the skin during washing. It is slow acting and particularly inhibits the growth of Gram-positive bacteria. These properties give additional safety in the use of surgical gloves when a small puncture during an operation may go unnoticed, but make it unsuitable as a single application skin preparation unless a quarter of an hour elapses before proceeding. The practice of using an alcohol rinse after preoperative hand washing with hexachlorophane compounds invalidates the action of hexachlorophane by washing it away since it is freely soluble in alcohol. In the early 1970s warnings were published concerning the possibility of toxic effects from absorption of hexachlorophane. Young babies are considered to be at greatest risk since they could be exposed to considerable amounts of the agent over the course of weeks of 'topping and tailing' and bathing. The use of hexachlorophane is now restricted to short-term use in some special hospital units.

pHisoHex contains 3% hexachlorophane and detergent.

Chlorhexidine. Chlorhexidine (Hibitane) is a complex synthetic organic compound of the diguanide group, active against a wide range of bacteria, including Gram-negative bacilli. Chlorhexidine in alcohol is an efficient, non-irritant skin germicide, and in aqueous solution is used for wound toilet and irrigation. Aqueous solutions are liable to contamination by organisms such as *Pseudomonas* sp.

Four per cent chlorhexidine detergent solution (Hibiscrub) is an effective skin cleansing agent which is widely used for hand-washing and preoperative skin preparation.

Quaternary ammonium compounds. These compounds, e.g. Roccal, Zephiran, Cetavlon, have very good detergent properties but are selective in action, being of limited use against Gram-negative bacteria and having no effect on tubercle bacilli, while proving effective against Gram-positive organisms such as staphylococci. The compounds include cationic, anionic and non-ionic solutions; if a cationic and an anionic solution are mixed the bacteriostatic activity of both is neutralized. They are also neutralized by soaps, hard water and various chemicals and have a peculiar adsorptive property. If the practice of moistening cotton wool balls by direct contact with the mouth of a bottle containing a quaternary ammonium is permitted, the solution in the bottle becomes progressively more inactive until only coloured water remains because the active agent is adsorbed on to the succession of wool balls. Not only will the remaining fluid be inactive but it will almost certainly become bacterially contaminated and cause infection when used for subsequent aseptic procedures.

Alcohols. *Ethyl alcohol* 70% is an effective skin germicide. Greater concentrations are less effective since water is essential to the transfer of the antiseptic across the bacterial cell wall.

Oxidizing Agents. *Hydrogen peroxide* is an antiseptic which liberates oxygen when in contact with organic material. The effervescence helps mechanically to loosen slough and pus in a wound but any remaining fluid will be plain water with no antiseptic property.

Nebulized hydrogen peroxide 10 vol. has been found to be a suitable means of decontaminating intermittent positive pressure ventilators (Whitby 1968).

Aldehydes. *Formaldehyde* 5% is an active, efficient disinfectant but has the disadvantage of a pungent smell and is very irritant to the skin, eyes and mucous membranes. *Glutaraldehyde* is as effective as formaldehyde without being irritant or voltatile. It is most active in an alkaline solution but since it is unstable in this form, the alkali has to be added to the glutaraldehyde shortly before use; e.g. Cidex 25%, an aqueous solution of glutaraldehyde, is diluted to 2% with an alkali, 0·3% NaCO, and can be used for the chemical sterilization of articles which will not withstand heat processing.

Gases

Formaldehyde gas. Total surface exposure to formaldehyde gas under conditions of controlled humidity, temperature and time exposure will destroy all vegetative bacteria, viruses and most spores. The best results are obtained with high concentrations of the gas, humidity above 60% and a temperature of not less than 18°C. The disadvantages of the gas are that it has a pungent smell, is irritant to eyes, skin and mucous membranes, and has poor properties of penetration and diffusion into fabrics or narrow tubes such as catheters.

Formaldehyde catheter 'sterilizing' ovens are unreliable and unsatisfactory; they should not be used (Department of Health and Social Security recommendation 1969).

This gas is occasionally used for terminal room disinfection and as a means of disinfecting mechanical apparatus such as patient ventilators. Extreme care in removing all traces of the gas by neutralizing with ammonia followed by very thorough airing of equipment before use is essential to patient safety.

Ethylene oxide gas. Ethylene oxide is a highly reactive colourless liquid with a boiling point of 10·7°C which is used in a gaseous state for sterilization of heat-sensitive materials. It has been used for many years to preserve foodstuffs and as an insecticide but only comparatively recently for medical purposes. The gas can be used at comparatively low temperatures, it does not corrode or damage a wide range of materials and, though much slower and less reliable than moist or dry heat, is a means of sterilizing equipment which would be ruined by both heat and ionizing radiation. The sterilizing process should be under skilled supervision since the efficiency of this agent is dependent on the correct balance of many interrelated factors.

1. Ethylene oxide penetrates and diffuses readily through porous loads, rubber and most plastics. A few plastics are adversely affected and acquire internal stresses after processing causing them to break in use. Penetration time, and therefore total sterilizing cycle time, varies according to the wrapping material as well as to the item contained in it. For example polyvinyl chloride films, aluminium laminates and films greater than 0·08 mm thick are relatively impermeable, penetration of Cellophane wrap is slow, but polythene and paper are easily and quickly permeated. Some metals (magnesium, zinc, tin) should not be exposed to the gas since they combine with ethylene oxide to form a sticky gel.

2. An effective cleaning process is of the greatest importance. As in every other sterilizing method, organic substances particularly proteins will prevent the essential contact between bacteria and the sterilizing agent. Bacteria suspended in salt solution are incorporated into the crystalline deposit on evaporation. This crystalline deposit is able to protect the bacteria from ethylene oxide and prevents their destruction. Both dirt and salt crystals remaining on equipment prevent sterilization by ethylene oxide.

3. It is thought that the gas has to be in solution on the bacterial cell surface to enable it to penetrate the cell wall and destroy the bacterium. Therefore both an adequate concentration of gas and sufficient moisture content throughout the load are also vital factors in achieving sterilization. It is important to avoid hot dry storage rooms and storage cupboards, the humidity in the preparation and packing areas should not be less than 50%. If the sterilizing load is a mixed one, containing perhaps two different plastics, metal, paper and rubber it is very difficult to ensure an even and adequate distribution of both gas and moisture since the materials

vary in density and moisture-retaining properties. It is even more difficult to establish a satisfactory but practical testing method.

4. Modern apparatus is designed to remove air from the loaded ethylene oxide sterilizer before the humidified gas is introduced. This facilitates even penetration of the load, eliminates the possibility of an explosive air/gas mixture and allows the use of pure ethylene oxide. Other apparatus which does not have a vacuum cycle commonly utilizes a mixture of 10% ethylene oxide and 90% of an inert gas such as carbon dioxide or freon to avoid the risk of an explosion.

5. Sterilization can be achieved at room temperature but requires a very long exposure time. Temperatures between 30° and 50°C are commonly used, the cycle times varying from 1 to 16 hours. The recommended gas concentration in and on the load is between 450 and 900 mg/litre.

6. Controlled conditions are essential for load packing, penetration and sterilization. They are equally essential for the safety of patients and staff handling packs and equipment after sterilization. Ethylene oxide takes time to diffuse out from materials, particularly rubber and plastics. The airing time required, even when a post vacuum is used, may be as long as 48 hours. Gas retained in equipment held in contact with the skin or mucous membrane will produce irritation and blistering.

Although the toxicity is defined as low and reversible the effects are unpleasant and in addition to adequate airing time, other safety measures such as good ventilation, correctly installed machine exhaust lines, and regular maintenance to detect and prevent leaks are necessary.

The following table gives examples of common situations and indicates appropriate disinfectants or antiseptics. It is not in any way a comprehensive list; solutions should be used in the strengths and dilutions recommended by the manufacturers.

Skin	Hands	4% Chlorhexidine detergent solution (Hibiscrub) Iodophors, e.g. Betadine, Wescodyne
	Preoperative preparation	Chlorhexidine in spirit (Hibitane) 4% Chlorhexidine detergent solution Ethyl alcohol 70% Tincture of iodine Iodophors
	Cleansing	Quaternary ammonium compounds, e.g. cetrimide, Roccal
Wound dressings	Gram-positive bacteria	Chlorhexidine
	Gram-negative bacteria	Eusol Electrolytic Sodium Hypochlorite (ESH)
	Slough and pus	Hydrogen peroxide 10 vol
	Burns	Silver nitrate 1%
Instruments and equipment which cannot be sterilized by heat or irradiation.		Formaldehyde 5% Glutaraldehyde, e.g. Cidex
Baby feed equipment		Electrolytic sodium hypochlorite, e.g. Milton
Kitchen hygiene		
Drinking water *Swimming baths*		Domestic bleach
Inanimate objects, surfaces *Floors, linen, etc.*		Phenolics and cresols, e.g. Hycolin, Sudol, Izal

FILTRATION

Pharmaceutical fluids and laboratory media which would be damaged by heat, ionizing radiation or chemicals are passed through filters to remove micro-organisms. The filters vary in material and design, e.g. unglazed porcelain, asbestos, glass fibre, collodion membranes, etc.

Air free from micro-organisms which may cause infection is required in operating theatres and other units for the protection of patients at high risk from infection. It is also a requirement where air is drawn into a sterile field such as the air inlet of an intravenous infusion set or an autoclave at the end of the sterilizing cycle. Protection from respiratory organisms may be achieved by the use of an efficient mask or a specially designed filter, e.g. a William's filter fitted into the circuit of a respirator.

Although the filters mentioned range from a wisp of cotton wool to a high efficiency particulate air filter (99·9% efficiency, 1 to 5 μm), if each is examined under a microscope the holes or the spaces between the fibres will be seen to be very much larger than the particles which they trap. Air passing through a filter induces a positive static charge in the fibres to which particles are attracted and held. If the fibres become moist the charge is earthed and the particles released, that is, a wet filter, e.g. a wet mask, allows organisms to pass through it.

8 Diagnostic Microbiology

Laboratory tests are prescribed by the clinician in charge of a patient for various reasons. For example, the test may be to find out which particular organism is causing an obvious infection, or it may be to confirm or to eliminate a specific site or system as the focus of infection. The patient may apparently have recovered from an infection and the test prescribed is to check that he is free from the causative organism, or a specimen may be one of a series sent at regular intervals to monitor progress.

The clinician may consult with the microbiologist about the suitability of certain tests, for expert interpretation of laboratory findings or for advice on antibiotic therapy; he frequently delegates to the nursing staff the responsibility for obtaining appropriate specimens.

The laboratory staff can only examine the material and information presented to them, and the diagnosis, management, or treatment of patients may depend on the results which they report back to the clinician. Collecting specimens at the correct time, using the correct technique and despatching them without delay to the designated laboratory is therefore of critical importance. If the material presented to the laboratory is of poor quality then the result of the test reported back to the clinician will be unreliable.

COLLECTION OF SPECIMENS FOR BACTERIOLOGICAL EXAMINATION

The objectives are:

1. To collect an adequate amount of tissue or fluid uncontaminated by further organisms from any other source

but preserving any organisms which may be present.

2. To ensure that the specimen is correctly identified by labelling, and sent to the laboratory with an accurately completed request form.

3. To transport the specimen from the patient to the laboratory safely and with the minimum of delay.

As a general rule the more material sent for examination, the greater the chance of isolating a causative organism. For example, it is preferable to send a few millilitres of pus aspirated with a sterile syringe and needle than to send a swab dipped in the pus.

Specimens are readily contaminated by poor techniques such as allowing urine to flow over the vulva before collecting it in the container, or by the use of unsterile equipment. Specimens should be collected in sterile laboratory containers, with the exception of faeces (clean container) and sputum (clean container free from respiratory organisms).

Ideally, samples should be collected before the commencement of antibiotic therapy. When it is necessary to test during a course of antibiotic, the specimen should be collected just before a dose is given.

Similarly when an antiseptic is used for cleaning or packing a wound or body cavity, a specimen should be collected at the commencement of the dressing procedure to minimize the risk of also collecting antiseptic. The presence of antibiotic or antiseptic in the specimen container may destroy organisms which are in fact active in the patient and this will affect laboratory tests. Such treatment should be noted on the request form accompanying the specimen.

It is important to ensure that every specimen is clearly identified by a label giving the name and location of the patient and the date. The accompanying request form should give any relevant data, e.g. a provisional diagnosis, pyrexia, wound infection, chemotherapy, as well as the patient's name, age, sex and location; it must be legible.

Culture plates, used in the ward for direct plating of eye swabs, should always be labelled with wax pencil, on the base and not the lid. This prevents errors if the lids are inadvertently exchanged during transit or processing. Plates are stored base uppermost for ease of handling.

The sooner specimens reach the laboratory the greater the chance of any organisms present surviving and being identified. With the exception of blood culture samples, which should be placed in a 37°C incubator, specimens which cannot be sent to the laboratory within a short time should be placed in a specimen refrigerator at 4°C. Some laboratories issue containers of sterile *transport medium* into which the tip of a swab stick may be broken by snapping it against the inside neck of the bottle, taking care not to contaminate this part of the shaft with the fingers. The purpose of transport medium is to preserve the organisms in the same condition and numbers as when present in the patient. It is effective for about 24 hours and should not be refrigerated or incubated.

Any specimen may contain pathogens. To avoid spreading organisms to other people or to the environment it is most important to avoid contamination of the outside of specimen containers and to ensure that they are securely closed and carefully handled. In the event of an *accidental spill* pour a small quantity of standard hospital disinfectant (e.g. Sudol or domestic bleach) on to the spilt material. Wearing a pair of disposable gloves and using paper towel or newspaper, mop up the spill. Contain the paper, debris and gloves within a waterproof bag for safe disposal. Wash the hands thoroughly.

If a specimen container leaks, not only are the porter and the laboratory staff at risk from accidental infection, but, since other contaminating bacteria can get into such a container even more easily than the specimen can leak out, a false answer to the test may be reported.

Delay *en route* to the laboratory is another factor which may affect the bacteria collected from a patient, particularly if the specimens are left in a warm place. For instance, a swab taken from a wound may dry out, causing the death of sensitive organisms, and this will result in a false negative report. Conversely, organisms multiply very fast in warm urine, so that the laboratory count of bacteria in a delayed specimen could be out of all

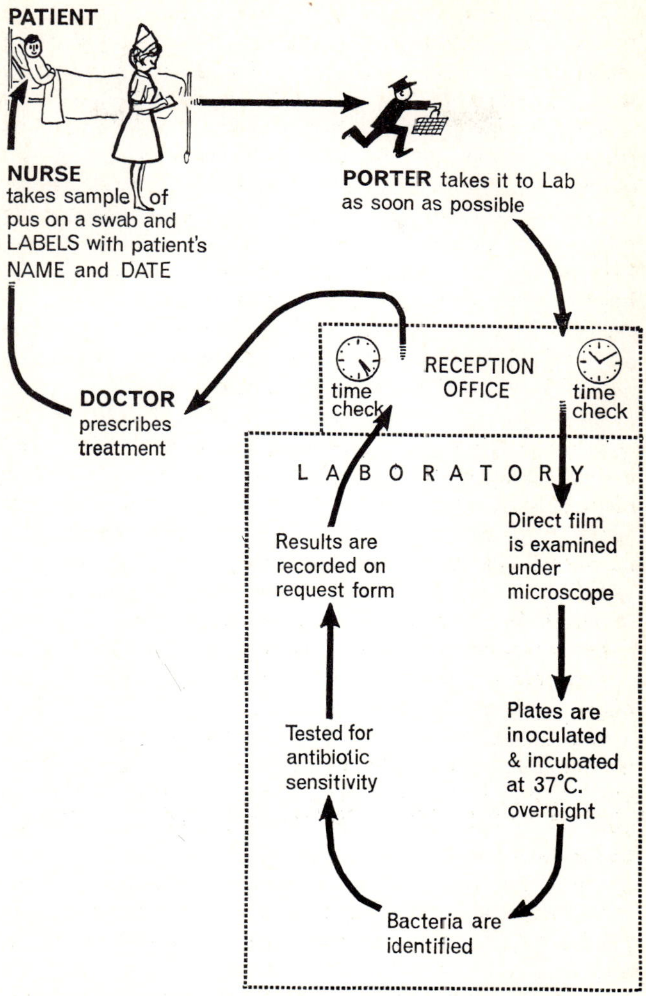

Fig. 20. *The sequence of laboratory identification of bacteria from infected material.*

proportion to that of the original specimen and a false positive report issued.

Nose and throat swabs. Swabs from the nose and throat are usually taken together, one swab for both tonsils and one for both nostrils; organisms causing sore throats are frequently carried in the nose and failure to take nose swabs may mean that the organisms here are missed.

The patient is placed facing a strong source of light and the tongue is depressed. The swab should never be removed from its sterile tube until everything is ready for taking the specimen. When taking a throat swab care should be taken to avoid touching the mouth or tongue with the swab, which should be gently rubbed over the pillars of the fauces and any area with a lesion or visible exudate.

When taking nasal swabs it is important to ensure that the swab reaches as far back as possible on each side; this can usually be done by tilting the patient's head back and using a gentle twisting movement. With babies and very young children wooden swab sticks are often too large to get into the nostrils and many hospitals supply fine wire swabholders covered with a tiny wisp of cotton wool. Care is needed to avoid damage to the delicate mucous membranes with these swabs. Swabs should be replaced in the sterile containers immediately, to avoid contamination with air organisms.

The normal healthy nose is virtually dry, therefore when routine screening is carried out to check staphylococcal carriage the swab should be moistened with sterile distilled water. In this case nasal swabs should be taken from the anterior nares and the swab directed upwards in the tip of the nose and gently rotated to collect any secretion.

Ear swabs. The same type of swab stick is used for ear swabs as for nose and throat swabs, and care should be taken that no antibiotics or other chemotherapeutic or antiseptic material has been used in the ear within three hours of taking the swab.

Wound swabs. Wound swabs are usually taken when a dressing is being changed; the same type of swab stick is used as for ear, nose and throat swabs. The swab should be rotated to collect as much pus or exudate as possible. It is then immediately replaced in the container or the tip is broken off within a bottle of sterile transport medium.

Puncture fluids. Large quantities of material for microbiological investigation are usually taken by syringe and may be transferred directly from this syringe to a sterile bottle. Pleural, ascitic and synovial fluids are collected into a sterile bottle containing an anticoagulant; 20–30 ml is an adequate amount for bacterial examination except when tuberculosis is suspected when the whole aspirate should be sent to the whole laboratory. Cerebrospinal fluid should be collected in dry sterile containers. Fluids requiring a cell count should be put into two sterile bottle appropriately labelled; the second one should be used for the count, since the first may contain extraneous blood cells introduced into the needle as it went through the tissues.

Sputum. The sputum is never free from organisms since material originating in the bronchi and alveoli has to pass through the pharynx and mouth which always have a normal commensal population of bacteria. The specimen containers need to be clean but not sterile, they must however be free from organisms of respiratory origin and most laboratories now use waxed paper or plastic disposable cartons with secure lids. Disinfectant should not be put in sputum pots which are to be sent for microbiological investigation.

Care should be taken that the material sent for investigation is in fact sputum and not saliva. Patients who have difficulty in bringing up phlegm should be encouraged to cough first thing in the morning. Patients with coughs usually have mucopurulent, or purulent flecks in the specimen. The specimen should be as large as possible and it is better to wait until an adequate specimen can be produced than to waste laboratory time on minute specimens of saliva. When the specimen has been coughed up the bacterial population alters in proportion rapidly; it is therefore important that the specimen should be sent to the laboratory immediately.

Specimens of sputum in cases of tuberculosis. The tubercle bacillus, *Mycobacterium tuberculosis,* may sometimes be thinly distributed in the sputum and a large quantity of material must therefore be submitted for examination on direct film and for cultures to be made. The bacillus is most likely to be present in the purulent flecks. It is usual to send three specimens of sputum taken on different days when looking for the tubercle bacillus; the results may not be available for six weeks or even longer, because cultures grow slowly. Patients with suspected pulmonary tuberculosis who are not producing any sputum usually have the stomach contents aspirated on three successive mornings before any food or liquid is taken. The total aspirate is sent to the laboratory as soon as possible.

Urine. Specimens of urine should normally be taken in the early morning when the urine has accumulated in the bladder over night: all specimens from one patient are then roughly comparable. If they are taken at other times the urine may sometimes be diluted due to a high fluid intake. Early morning specimens are not, of course, possible in out-patient clinics, but they should be the rule for in-patients. In examination for tubercle bacilli in the urine, where the organisms are likely to be very scanty, the whole of the specimen should be sent in a sterile bottle.

Specimens of urine from male patients should be 'mid-stream specimens'; that is to say, after the skin surrounding the urethral meatus has been cleansed the patient micturates and the middle portion of the stream is collected directly into a sterile container to avoid contamination of the specimen with organisms normally present on the skin.

The collection of an uncontaminated mid-stream specimen from a female patient is not easy and should be carried out under nursing supervision when possible. The external genitalia and then the urethral meatus should be carefully cleansed. The patient micturates with the labia separated, and the middle portion of the stream is collected directly into a wide-mouthed sterile container.

A urine specimen from a patient who has an indwelling catheter should be aspirated, with a sterile syringe and needle, through the catheter wall. If the catheter has no aspiration insert and is too rigid for safe puncture, the drainage tubing insert may be used. It is much less satisfactory to collect the specimen from the end of the catheter. The sample should never be taken from the drainage bag.

Urine specimens should reach the laboratory within 1 hr or be refrigerated at 4°C until transported so that the numbers and types of different bacteria can be accurately assessed.

Faeces. Specimens of stools for examination should be sent in clean but unsterile cartons which may be subsequently burnt. Some bacteriologists allow rectal swabs for the detection of the organisms causing food poisoning or dysentery. These swabs are of the same type as those used for wounds and the nose and throat, and care should be taken to pass the swab through the anus right into the rectum. It is advisable to send a specimen of stool as well if this is available so that the amount of pus, blood and mucus and the consistency of the specimen can then be seen.

Specimens of stools for parasites. Segments of *tapeworm* can be seen with ease in any specimen of stool and the worm will continue to grow and shed segments unless the head is dislodged; it is therefore important to search for this in every specimen passed by the patient after treatment. Stool specimens should be strained through fine black material under a running tap, the tapeworm segments will be retained and can be sent to the laboratory for identification of the species and for confirmation of the presence of the head.

Many intestinal worms shed their *ova* into the faeces; they can only be seen microscopically and a fresh specimen of stool should be sent to the laboratory in a waxed carton. Threadworms lay their ova on the perianal skin; swabs of this area should therefore be taken as the ova will not be seen in stool specimens. The sticky side of transparent Sellotape is used for this purpose and is pressed on to the skin of the perianal area, in the early morning and before defaecation. The Sellotape should then be placed adhesive side down on to a glass slide which is sent to the laboratory.

Specimens of stool for amoebae. The parasites of amoebic dysentery, *Entamoeba histolytica,* exist in a free-living motile form and in the form of non-motile cysts. Both forms are characteristic in their fresh state and a diagnosis of amoebic dysentery can be made from a fresh specimen of stool. The free-living form, however, becomes non-motile very easily in older specimens when the temperature has fallen, and both forms are more difficult to recognize when they are dead. It is therefore essential that specimens of stool for amoebae should be sent to the laboratory as soon as they are passed and should be looked at immediately. It may be necessary to examine many specimens before the amoebae are seen.

Eye swabs. Either a wire loop or cottonwool-covered wooden stick should be used. Rub gently over the conjunctiva in the lower conjuctival sac, taking care to hold the swab parallel to the cornea and to avoid contamination by touching the lids. Conjunctival swabs should be inoculated on to an agar plate at the bedside as the lysozyme normally present in tears is antibacterial in action.

Purulent conjunctivitis in babies may be due to the gonococcus, which is a very delicate organism and may be killed if the swabs are allowed to dry or get cold. In some hospitals it is a routine procedure in cases of purulent conjunctivitis, to take two swabs. One of these swabs is broken into a bottle of transport medium, the other swab can be sent to the laboratory together with this bottle so that direct films of the pus can be stained.

Vaginal swabs. Special charcoal-impregnated swabs should be used and the specimens should be taken from as high in the vaginal vault as possible after introduction of a speculum to separate the walls. If *Trichomonas* infection is suspected the swab should be broken off in Fineberg's medium. Other cervical, urethral and vaginal swabs should be broken off in Stuart's transport medium. Specimens may also be taken with a teated pipette contained in a test tube.

Blood cultures. Samples of blood are usually taken by the medical staff and are used for direct isolation of a pathogenic organism in a case of septicaemia, and for detection of antibodies in the serum; in either case the specimens should be taken with full aseptic precautions; a dry, sterile syringe is used.

Success or failure in isolating organisms present in the blood stream is largely dependent upon taking the specimen at the right time and putting it into suitable medium for cultivation, and in this the nursing staff can give valuable assistance.

The clinician will tell the microbiologist what organism he thinks may be present, the microbiologist will choose the correct medium, and the blood is put directly into one of more bottles of this fluid. Organisms are most likely to be present in the blood stream in the greatest number when the temperature is at its highest, so that the most favourable time for taking a blood culture is at the peak of the temperature. The ward sister's knowledge of the patient's previous temperature range will help in predicting when this is likely to be, and it is her duty to keep a watch on his temperature and inform the medical officer or the laboratory when this is rising. With all requests for blood cultures certain information should be sent to the laboratory:

1. The time the blood culture was taken and the patient's temperature at that time.
2. The length of time the patient has been ill.
3. Any inflammatory lesions the patient may have, e.g. pneumonia, septic wound, urinary infection and the microbiology of these lesions if known.
4. Any chemotherapeutic treatment the patient may be having, and when he had his last dose. (Chemotherapeutic drugs for this purpose would include antibiotics.)

Serum for detection of antibodies. For this investigation 10 ml of blood should be taken into a dry tube or bottle containing no anticoagulant, and allowed to clot.

Specific antibodies do not appear in the serum for several days. It is the usual procedure to take blood at the beginning of a disease and then again after 10 days; the specimens are examined together in the laboratory. An increase in the amount of antibodies in the second specimen will be an indication of continued stimulation by the organism which must therefore be present in the patient. By comparing two specimens more information is gained, although single samples are sometimes helpful.

It is important that samples are accompanied by full details of:

1. The clinical history.
2. The length of time the patient has been ill.
3. Any history of a previous attack of the disease, with dates.
4. Any history of immunization.

THE COLLECTION OF MATERIAL FOR DIAGNOSIS OF FUNGAL INFECTIONS

Hair. Samples of broken and infected hairs should be removed with forceps and sent to the laboratory in a clean sealed envelope or suitably dry specimen container so that the base of the hair can be examined and cultured. Some fungi fluoresce in ultra-violet light and a lamp may be used to identify infected hairs.

Nails. The whole thickness of the nail or deep scrapings should be sent in a dry container to the laboratory.

Skin lesions. The skin should be cleaned with alcohol. Epidermal scales scraped from the active edge of a lesion or the roof of any vesicles should be sent to the laboratory in a dry container.

Other specimens. Sputum, ear swabs, body fluids and curettings are collected in the same way as specimens for bacteriological examination.

THE COLLECTION OF SPECIMENS FOR VIROLOGICAL INVESTIGATION

Virus laboratories usually supply special transport media and should be consulted before specimens are taken. In addition to the patient data sent with a specimen for bacteriological examination (p.86) the virologist will require the date of the onset of the illness, and the patient's immunization record particularly of any inoculation within one month.

If the specimen cannot be delivered to the laboratory within 1 hr of collection it should be refrigerated at 4°C.

When viral disease is suspected several different specimens may be taken.

Central nervous system disease: Cerebrospinal fluid, brain, blood, faeces, throat swabs or washings.

Respiratory disease: Sputum, throat swabs or washings.

Eye disease: Conjunctival swabs or scrapings.

Skin lesions: Vesicle or pustule fluid in capillary tubes, air-dried slides from scrapings of macules or papules.

Serological tests will also be undertaken, for which 5–10 ml of clotted blood are required. At least two blood samples are collected, the first as soon as possible after the onset of illness, the second two to three weeks later, so that the antibody levels (titre) can be assessed and compared. A rising antibody titre is diagnostic of infection by the relevant virus.

ISOLATION OF THE CAUSATIVE ORGANISM FROM INFECTED MATERIAL

The microbiologist identifies an organism in material which is sent to him by a number of tests which have been designed to tell him a series of facts:

1. Morphology or size and shape of the organism and its staining properties.
2. Conditions for growth.
3. Cultural characteristics.
4. Biochemical tests.
5. Resistance.
6. Serological tests.
7. Pathogenicity tests in experimental animals.

Morphology of the Organism

The organisms present in any specimen sent to the microbiologist are examined to determine their size, shape and other specific characteristics. They may be from 0·3 μm to 14 μm in length (1 μm = 0·001 mm). They may be round, rod-shaped or spiral. They may grow in pairs, in clusters or in chains, and a given culture may contain organisms of irregular size and shape. They may possess flagella or may bear spores. To make them readily visible they are stained with various dyes in different ways to distinguish them according to the effects of various staining processes.

Staining. The bacterial kingdom can be roughly divided into two by the action of a staining technique called *Gram's method,* which consists of staining the cells with a basic dye, methyl violet, and afterwards treating with iodine. The film stain is then decolorized with alcohol or acetone, until no more is removed. The organisms are subsequently counterstained with a red contrasting coloured dye, e.g. safranin. Gram-positive organisms are those which retain the methyl violet and appear purple under the microscope. Gram-negative ones are those which do not retain the dye and are stained red by the counterstain. Hence bacteria are divided into Gram-positive and Gram-negative groups and this grouping, together with the bacterial shape, cocci, bacilli or very short ovoid organisms called coccobacilli, gives the bacteriologist a start in his identification.

The tubercle bacillus (*Mycobacterium tuberculosis*) and related organisms are stained only with difficulty by Gram's stain, but can be reliably stained by using hot, strong carbol fuchsin, which stain is impossible to remove with acid and alcohol. This is the basis of the *Ziehl-Neelsen* stain and the organisms so stained are said to be 'acid-alcohol fast'.

Organisms which are able to move by means of flagella or hair-like structures which may be placed in various positions on the bacterial body can be stained by special techniques only. The spirochaetes such as *Treponema pallidum,* the organism responsible for syphilis, are capable of movement by bending their spiral bodies and the rate and character of the movement is characteristic. Some organisms such as the pneumococcus are surrounded by a clear capsule which can be demonstrated by special stains.

Condition of Growth

It is the usual procedure, when endeavouring to isolate an organism, to put infected material into a sterile mixture containing nutriment which is suitable to encourage the growth of likely organisms. The foodstuffs are called 'culture media' and many have a meat infusion, like clear soup, as a basis, which is put into sterile bottles; a swab previously dipped in infected material is broken into one of these. The meat infusion may be mixed with hot melted agar-agar, poured into flat dishes called Petri dishes or into screw-capped bottles, set aslant, and allowed to set. Infected material is spread on the surface of these using a fine wire loop.

To encourage the growth of various organisms certain other substances can be added to the basic medium either to enrich it, or to make it selective. For example, amino acids, proteins in the form of serum, plasma or whole blood, or vitamins may be used as enrichments.

Selective media are those which contain substances known to inhibit certain organisms or groups of organisms. They are also useful in the detection of pathogenic organisms from material such as stools and throat swabs, both of which are normally full of organisms. If unselective enriched media are used, the normal non-pathogenic organisms may overgrow the sparse pathogens and make their detection difficult. In practice there are selective media for many species and certain media have become routine for primary inoculation of material from most sites.

Cultural Characteristics

In order to ascertain the cultural characteristics of an organism, infected material is introduced into suitable fluid and solid media. On the latter it is spread thinly over the whole plate with a wire loop, which is sterilized in a flame before and after use. The inoculated media are then put into incubators adjusted to a constant temperature. In medical microbiology 37°C is the temperature of primary incubation, because the majority of human pathogens have this as their optimum temperature.

Many organisms, such as the staphylococcus or the diphtheria bacillus, grow best in an atmosphere containing oxygen; they grow well therefore in air and are said to be aerobic organisms, Some, such as the gonococcus, the organism causing gonorrhoea, grow best in an atmosphere containing carbon dioxide, and for isolation of this organism from an infected patient the inoculated

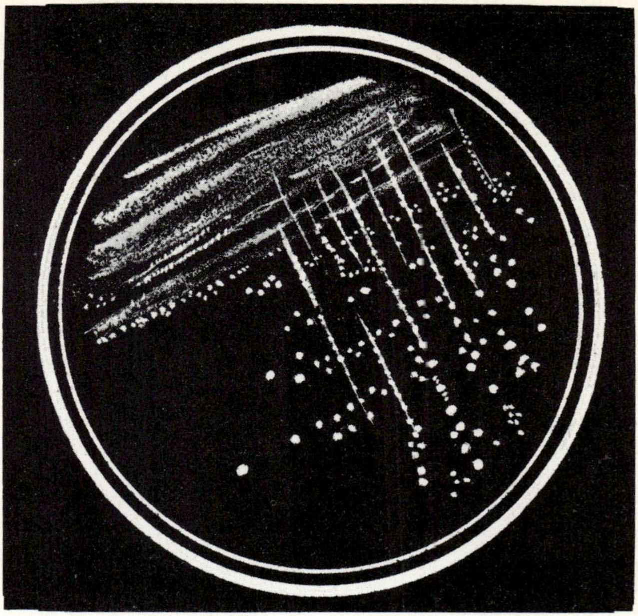

Fig. 21. *Colonies on a plate spread by the method of parallel streaks. A small portion of the material to be examined is spread over the surface by successive parallel strokes of a wire loop.*

plates are put into a tin which contains 5% carbon dioxide and are put in the incubator. Other organisms, such as *Clostridium tetani,* cannot grow where there is free oxygen, and to grow these organisms conditions must be made anaerobic by placing the plates in a tin or jar, partially evacuating the air which is then replaced with hydrogen. The hydrogen is combined with the residual oxygen to produce completely anaerobic conditions. These are strictly anaerobic organisms, but there are some facultative anaerobes, that is to say they are equipped with enzymes which allow them to utilize either aerobic or anaerobic respiration. Organisms such as streptococci have this ability.

It is usual to leave the plates undisturbed in the

incubator overnight (18 to 24 hours) before looking for growth. Some organisms grow slowly and often no growth is visible to the naked eye at this time. With other organisms, along the lines of inoculation there will be heaped colonies of growing organisms, ranging from 0·1 mm to 4 mm in diameter. These colonies, each containing many organisms, all of the same kind, have developed by division of the initial ones put on with the loop. Their size, shape, colour, consistency and effect on the surrounding medium are all of importance and characteristic of the species. Instead of isolated colonies the organisms may have spread in a film all over the plate; organisms which do this are those which are highly motile, that is capable of movement in the thin film of water which covers the surface of the plate.

Biochemical Tests

Certain biochemical tests have been found useful to differentiate various bacteria. The majority of these tests are designed to detect the presence of enzymes in the organisms which bring about a specific chemical reaction. The *Shigella* group of organisms, those causing dysentery, are morphologically and culturally identical, but can be differentiated by the different carbohydrates which they can break down by enzyme action, so as to use them as a source of energy. If these organisms are grown in medium containing mannitol as a source of carbohydrate, certain of them can break this down, and the breakdown products will be acid in reaction. If, therefore, an indicator is added which will show acid production by its change in colour, this change indicates the ability to ferment mannitol and tells the bacteriologist that this organism may be *Shigella sonnei,* or one of the *Shigella flexneri* organisms, if other reactions also fit in with what is known of these organisms.

Some organisms are soluble in bile; a *Pneumococcus* may be differentiated from a viridans type of *Streptococcus* by tests making use of this principle.

The ability to break down and use starch is a

characteristic which differentiates the one strain of diphtheria bacillus from the other members of the genus *Corynebacterium,* and is a useful differentiating test. The ability to form indole in a medium containing tryptophan is a characteristic of many non-pathogenic Gram-negative intestinal organisms. There are many other examples used diagnostically, all reflecting fundamental metabolic processes which have by experience been found useful in differentiating one organism from another.

Resistance

The resistance of an organism to temperature, drying, acid, antiseptics, dyes, chemotherapeutic agents and antibodies, is a help in diagnosis as well as a help in treatment and prevention of spread. As we have already seen, those organisms which have not the power of forming spores are relatively less resistant to heat than the spore-bearing organisms. Some haemolytic streptococci will be killed if kept at 60°C for 30 minutes; certain other streptococci, may be differentiated by a heat resistance test, since they withstand 60°C for 30 minutes. Very heat resistant spores bearing organisms such as *Bacillus anthracis* will withstand 100°C for a considerable time.

The sensitivity of various organisms to the antibiotics, although it may be of value in differentiating strains, is of more value as a guide to therapy.

Serology

An organism isolated from infected material contains numerous antigens; if these are mixed with serum containing known specific antibodies prepared by injection of a known organism into an experimental animal, and the unknown organism reacts with the specific antiserum, the antigens in the unknown organism must be the same as or closely related to those which were used to immunize the experimental animal. Antigen–antibody reactions are used a great deal in bacteriology, the union of antigen with antibody being associated with an

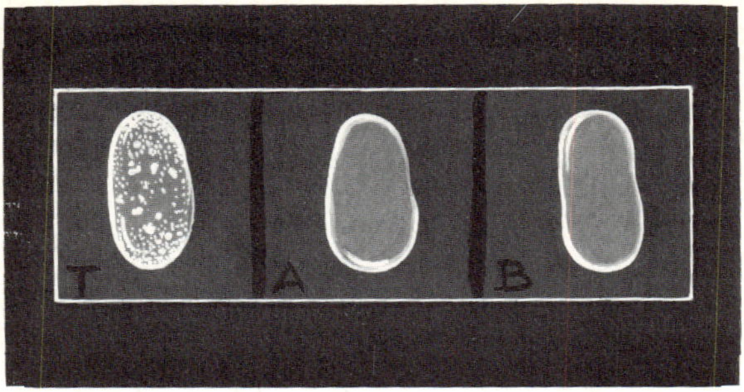

Fig. 22. *Slide agglutination seen by naked eye. A culture of bacteria from a suspected typhoid carrier has been mixed with drops of antisera prepared against* Salmonella typhi *(T),* Salm. paratyphi *(A), and* Salm. paratyphi *(B). It has been agglutinated by T but not by A or B. Therefore the organism is identified as the typhoid bacillus.*

altered physical state of the mixture such as a clumping of red blood cells, which enables it to be seen. Use is also made of these reactions, as we have seen before, in detecting unknown antibodies in the patient's serum, the serum being mixed with known organisms acting as antigens. This principle forms the basis of the Widal test for enteric fever (Fig. 22).

Inoculation of Infected Material into Laboratory Animals

Some infectious agents cannot be cultured on artificial media, and their presence can only be detected by producing the disease in an experimental animal which is known to be susceptible. Tissues from the animal may show changes typical of the disease. For example, when tubercle bacilli cannot be found in the urine, tuberculosis may sometimes be produced in a guinea-pig by injection with some of the infected fluid.

These are the means, then, by which the bacteriologist is able to identify organisms present in the material which is sent to him, but it will be obvious that this identification

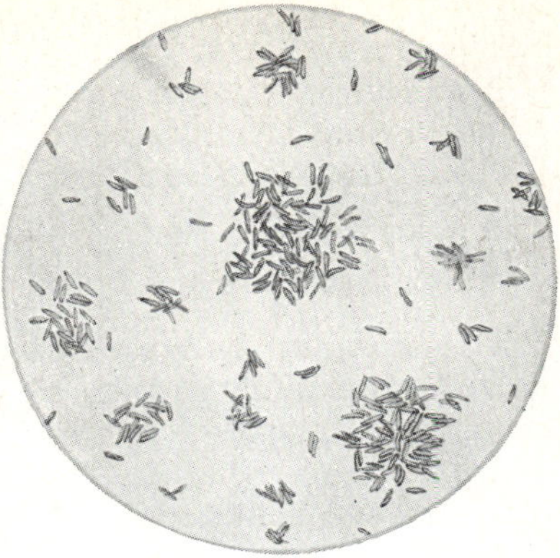

Fig. 23. *Agglutination as seen under the microscope.*

is bound to take time. In rare cases the organisms can be seen in direct films of the material and their appearance will be diagnostic. More commonly 18 hr are necessary for the organisms to be grown on media and only then can the various differential tests be applied.

In specimens taken from sites which are normally inhabited by organisms, such as the respiratory tract, the stools, and lesions involving the skin, the bacterial flora will be mixed and before identification can begin the organisms must be separated and isolated in pure culture.

THE DEMONSTRATION OF ANTIBODIES IN PATIENT'S SERUM

The diagnosis of infectious disease by demonstrating the presence of antibodies in the patient's serum is discussed under Immunity in Chapter 5; it is as well to note that the inference to be drawn from the presence of specific antibodies in a patient's serum is limited. All that can be deduced is that the patient has at some time been subjected to the specific antigen under test. A present attack of the disease is best diagnosed by taking repeated samples of serum and showing that these contain an increase in antibody content or 'titre'.

HYPERSENSITIVITY TESTS SUGGESTING A PREVIOUS DOSE OF A PATHOGENIC ORGANISM

Hypersensitivity reactions may be: (*a*) Immediate, when they are an allergic response of the body to certain foreign proteins and occur in the cellular structures affected, e.g. hay fever. (*b*) Delayed, when the response is dependent on immunologically activated lymphocytes reaching the site of entry of the antigen. The delay is due to the fact that the lymphocytes have to migrate to this site, e.g. tuberculin test.

This reaction of sensitivity is the basis of the tuberculin test. A positive reaction does not necessarily mean that the patient has the active disease at the time of the test, but that he has at some previous date had a dose of the antigen. The diagnostic value of a positive tuberculin test is therefore limited. Many people have a primary dose of tuberculosis in their childhood or adolescence, which they overcome without difficulty and with no clinical symptoms, and the majority of adults are therefore tuberculin positive.

NON-SPECIFIC TESTS

There are certain tests which have been found by experience to be positive in certain diseases, although the reasons are unknown. These tests are mainly antigen–antibody reactions. The patient's serum in certain diseases contains an antibody which reacts with an antigen which did not stimulate its production, that is to say, one other than the infecting agent. It is probable that this infecting agent and the test antigen are, however, chemically and and antigenically related. This happens in some circumstances with the *Salmonella* group of diseases.

Weil-Felix reaction. An attack of typhus stimulates the production of antibodies which react with a certain strain of *Proteus,* and in this test the *Proteus* organism is used as the antigen. More specific tests, using the typhus *Rickettsia* itself, are replacing this test.

Cold agglutinins. The infective agent or agents responsible for virus pneumonia have never been isolated, so that specific antigen–antibody reactions are not possible. It has been shown, however, that certain patients with this disease develop in their serum antibodies which agglutinate human group O cells at a low temperature. This is of some help in diagnosis.

There are many examples, too numerous to mention, of non-specific serological tests used in diagnosis of past or present infectious diseases, and as more is known of the antigenic and chemical nature of the infective agents, the reasons for the phenomena may become apparent.

THE LABORATORY REPORT

Features Described in the Report

Macroscopy. The gross appearance of the specimen received by the laboratory may be important information to the clinician assessing the report, e.g. *Staphylococcus aureus* present in saliva may be due to nasal carriage of the organism, but the same organism in a true specimen of sputum is most likely to be due to severe chest infection.

Microscopy. Information is gained from looking at prepared slides under the microscope, such as the presence of cells, casts or crystals, yeasts or fungi, parasites or their ova. It is usual, when tuberculosis is suspected, for the reports to state 'ZN positive' or 'ZN negative' with 'further report to follow' because of the time required to obtain a definitive answer on culture. A negative Ziehl-Neelsen test does not mean that the patient is not tuberculous. It means that tubercle bacilli were not seen in the part of the single specimen examined. A positive report usually means that there were large numbers of tubercle bacilli present, i.e. the patient has active disease.

Culture. This is the information gained from culturing the organism and its identification.

1. The organism is named, e.g. *Streptococcus* (the family name). This may be followed by the abbreviation sp(p). = species, or a further identification of the member of the family, e.g. *Streptococcus faecalis* or *Streptococcus pyogenes*.
2. The growth of the organism may be described in terms of quality, e.g. heavy or moderate, or it may be described quantitively, e.g. the number of bacteria per litre of urine, expressed as $> 10^8$/litre.
3. The laboratory may report on the presence or absence of a particular organism only, because the clinician does not require any other information. This is described as a screening test and the report states, for example 'No *Salmonella* sp. isolated'.

Antibiotic sensitivity. The sensitivity of a pathogen to a range of antibiotic is reported as a guide to the clinician if he considers that the patient requires antibiotic therapy. s = sensitive, r = resistant.

Serology. The dosage of certain antibiotics, e.g. gentamicin, is controlled in some patients by the estimation of serum levels of the drug. Trough and peak levels are usually reported in μg/ml. Antibody titres may be reported in figures, e.g. 1 in 200, or may be interpreted by the microbiologists, e.g. 'shows a significant rise in titre' (a titre is the highest dilution at which antibody is detected).

The Use of Laboratory Reports

Laboratory reports should only be interpreted with knowledge of the clinical condition of the patient. The fact that a pathogen and antibiotic sensitivities are reported does not necessarily imply that the patient must be given therapy; he may already be recovering from the infection. The fact that no organism was isolated does not necessarily mean that the site was sterile; it could be the result of poor technique in obtaining the specimen.

On the other hand, reports may contribute towards establishing a diagnosis, the prescription of treatment or further surgery, or they may be used in series as a measure of a patient's progress. Reports give information on which to base decisions concerning the nursing care of patients, the pattern of the day's work in a ward, the movement and grouping of patients and measures necessary to contain, or to prevent the spread of infection.

9 A Guide to Common Pathogenic Bacteria

The aim of this chapter is to present some outstanding facts about common organisms which the nurse may use for quick reference when she meets them in laboratory reports.

Most of the organisms have two or even three names, and in the pages that follow the present international name used by microbiologists is given first, followed by the common names used in Britain before the international nomenclature was adopted. Abbreviations which are readily understood by those without professional bacteriological experience have been used in preference to the short correct version. For example, *Salm.* is used instead of *S.* for *Salmonella* and *Esch.* for *E.* meaning *Escherichia.*

THE MAIN DIVISIONS OF MICRO-ORGANISMS

The population of the microbiological world can be grouped into six divisions:

1. Non-branching organisms stained by crystal violet + iodine (Gram-positive) (staining, see p. 98).
2. Non-branching organisms not stained by crystal violet + iodine (Gram-negative).
3. Branching organisms, Gram-positive and Gram-negative.
4. Organisms stained by the Ziehl Neelsen technique (acid-fast).

5. Some spirochaetes which are often difficult to stain by the techniques mentioned above.
6. Organisms only seen inside stained cells (viruses and rickettsiae) or by means of an electron microscope.

1. GRAM-POSITIVE DIVISION

STREPTOCOCCUS

Oval cocci in pairs or chains like strings of beads. Found everywhere. Many inhabit mucous membranes of man and animals, including mouth, upper respiratory tract and intestine. Many live in food, especially milk and dairy products, where they are found with the *Lactobacillus*. Some kinds discolour or destroy red blood cells and are called 'haemolytic streptococci'.

PATHOGENIC

- β-haemolytic *Streptococcus*
  - *Str. pyogenes* (Group A) cause of **tonsillitis, scarlet fever, acute nephritis, acute rheumatic fever, puerperal fever, wound infection, erysipelas, cellulitis**
  - Lancefield groups B C G
- *Str. pneumoniae* (pneumococcus) cause of **primary pneumonia, meningitis, peritonitis**

POTENTIALLY PATHOGENIC

- *Str. faecalis* (Lancefield Group D)
- *Str. viridans* may cause **sub-acute bacterial endocarditis**

HARMLESS TO MAN
Hundreds of strains

Grouping of Streptococci

Beta-haemolytic streptococci are grouped by identification of specific chemical antigens into 14 Lancefield groups

A–O. Groups A, C and G are usually responsible for human streptococcal infections. Group A is the most virulent and is responsible for the majority of these infections. During an outbreak of streptococcal infection it may be necessary to distinguish between two or more Group A strains. This is done by serological tests which subdivide Group A strains into about 40 different Griffith types.

STAPHYLOCOCCUS

Spherical cocci in clusters like grapes. Found on mucous membranes, skin, and as a contaminant in air and soil.

PATHOGENIC

Staphylococcus aureus, or coagulase-positive staphylococcus, sometimes called *Staph. pyogenes*. Usually enters through the skin, but may enter through mucous membranes. Spread by human carriers and found in about 50% of people, especially hospital staff. Cause of all kinds of **abscesses, boils, carbuncles, whitlows, styes, breast abscess, pemphigus neonatorum, infected wounds, pneumonia, and one form of food poisoning**

HARMLESS

Staphylococcus epidermis, Staphylococcus albus and *Staphylococcus citreus*. Coagulase-negative, found in nose and on the skin, and in the environment

Typing of Coagulase-positive Staphylococci

Coagulase-positive staphylococci can be typed and identified by the effect of staphylococcal bacteriophage upon them. Bacteriophages are highly specific viruses not pathogenic to man, which attack and destroy susceptible bacteria. This typing is important to the infection control team; there are many types of *Staphylococcus* and the bacteriologist tries to find out which particular type is the cause of cross-infection in an outbreak. Swabs may be taken from staff and patients to identify the troublesome strain and to try to trace its spread from patient to patient. Sometimes the source may be the nose of an individual whose wound becomes infected, an example of bacteria which are saprophytic in one situation and pathogenic in another. This is autoinfection.

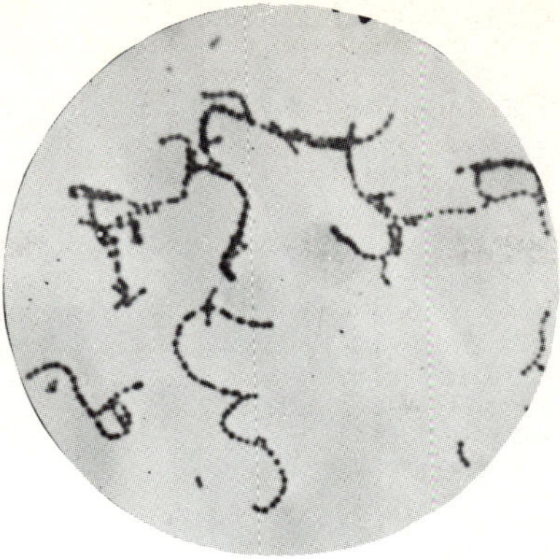

Fig. 24. *Culture smear of* Streptococcus pyogenes *showing the characteristic chain arrangement of streptococci (× 1000).*

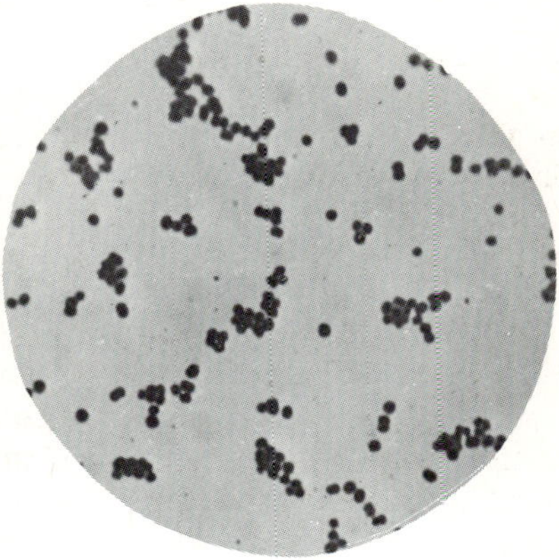

Fig. 25. *Culture smear of* Staphyloccus aureus *showing characteristic clumping (×1000).*

CORYNEBACTERIUM

Rod-shaped. Found on skin and mucous membranes particularly of the respiratory tract.

PATHOGENIC	HARMLESS
C. diphtheriae (diphtheria bacillus, or Klebs-Loeffler bacillus). Usual portal of entry is the upper respiratory tract, but occasionally the vagina, the skin or the conjunctiva. Spread by human carriers. Cause of **diphtheria**	*C. hofmannii, C. xerosis* and other diphtheroids, commonly found as skin commensals

C. diphtheriae is distinguished from the harmless members of the group by biochemical tests, but principally by exotoxin-production, which may be demonstrated by guinea pig inoculation. The Schick test is an intradermal test with toxin which determines a patient's susceptibility to diphtheria.

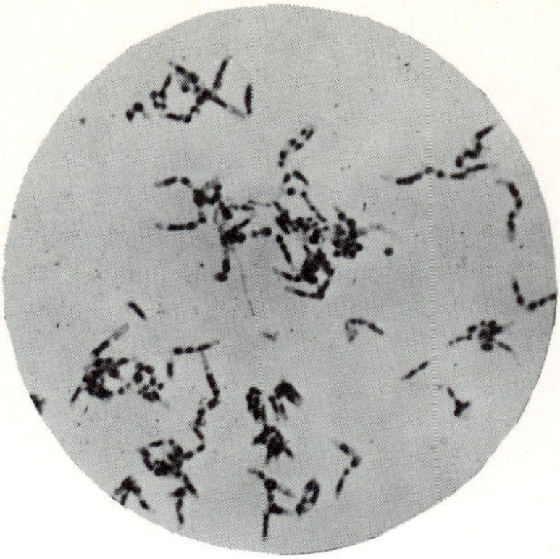

Fig. 26. *Culture smear of* Corynebacterium diphtheriae *showing characteristic arrangement and uneven staining (× 1000).*

CLOSTRIDIUM

Rods with spores which are wider than the parent organism, shaped like spindle, key or tennis racket. Found in the intestinal tract of man and animals and, of course, in soil. Anaerobe. Many members are harmless (*Clostridium sporogenes*) and even the pathogenic members may not cause disease unless the organisms or spores are carried into wounds, or tissues where conditions are exactly suitable for growth and toxin production.

PATHOGENIC

Cl. tetani, or *Bacillus tetani.* Produces exotoxin when carried into wounds. This poisons the anterior horn cell of the spinal cord thus affecting the motor nerves, producing an effect not unlike strychnine, resulting in the disease **tetanus**	*Cl. welchii (perfringens)* or *Bacillus welchii.* Produces toxin when carried into wounds involving muscle with damaged blood supply. The muscle infection produced is known as **gas gangrene.** Other important gas gangrene producers are *Cl. septique* and *Cl. oedematiens*	*Cl. botulinum,* or *Bacillus botulinum.* Produces toxin in tinned, potted or semi-cooked food, usually vegetable. The poisoned food when eaten causes acute toxaemia characterized by paralysis of the cranial motor nerves and of the diaphragm which is known as **botulism**

Certain strains of *Cl. perfringens* are associated with a mild form of food poisoning.

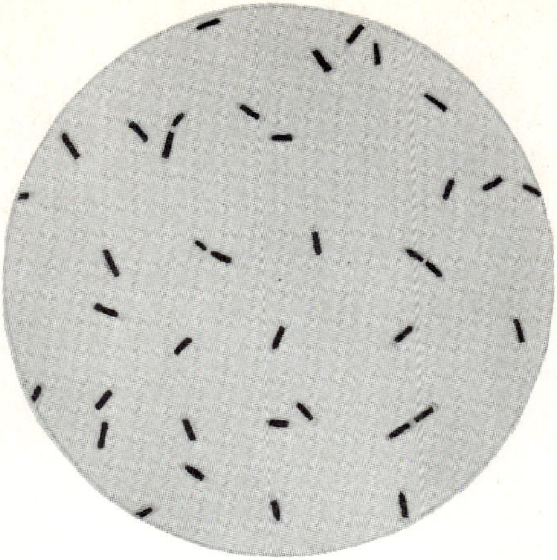

Fig. 27. Clostridium welchii *showing characteristic brick-shaped bacilli (× 1000).*

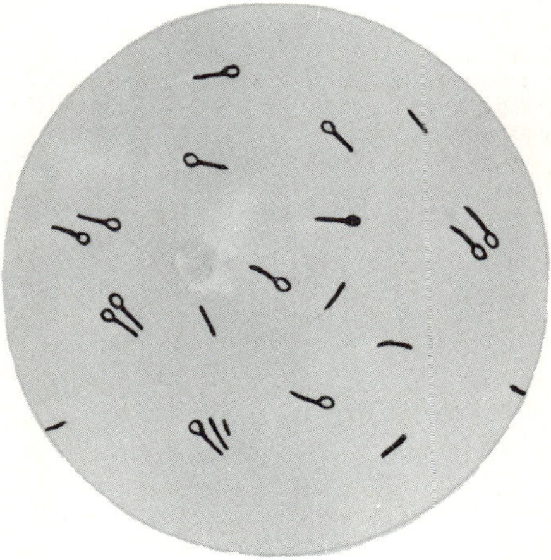

Fig. 28. *Diagram showing delicate rod-shaped* Clostridium tetani, *with many round terminal spores, characteristically drum-shaped (× 1200).*

BACILLUS

Large rods with spores which do not swell the organisms. Spores very resistant to heat and other physical and chemical agents. Aerobe. Found in air, soil, water, dust, wool, hair, carcases.

PATHOGENIC	HARMLESS
B. anthracis, or anthrax bacillus. Enters through the skin, spores inhaled into the lungs or swallowed. Spread by animals and animal products, such as hides, hair, wool, infected carcases and bedding. Cause of **anthrax**	*B. subtilis*. Very widely distributed in dust

B. anthracis is distinguished from the harmless members of the group by biochemical tests and pathogenicity tests in animals.

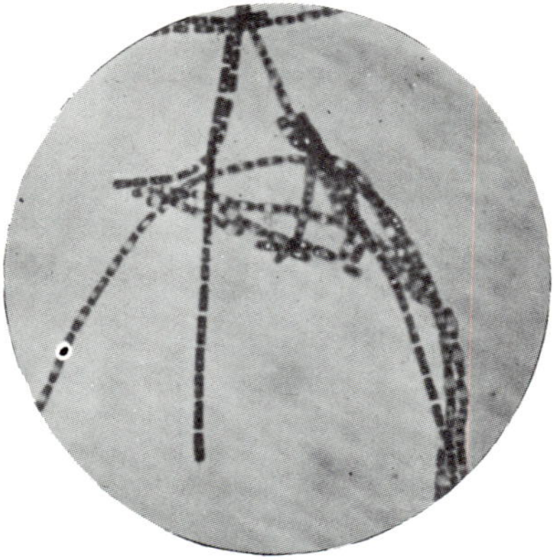

Fig. 29. *Culture smear of* Bacillus anthracis *showing chain formation and many spores (× 900).*

CANDIDA

Candida albicans (Monilia) is an oval, yeast-like *fungus* which is strongly Gram-positive. In cultures and in tissues it frequently grows filamentous threads in addition to the usual budding yeast forms. It is found in the normal flora of mucous membranes in the mouth, intestinal tract and vagina. Occasionally, often in association with another pathological condition, it becomes the dominant strain and infection results. Such infections are generally local, but very rarely they produce progressive systemic disease. This organism is resistant to all antibacterial antibiotics and flourishes in patients being so treated. Commonly transmitted from patient to patient in hospitals.

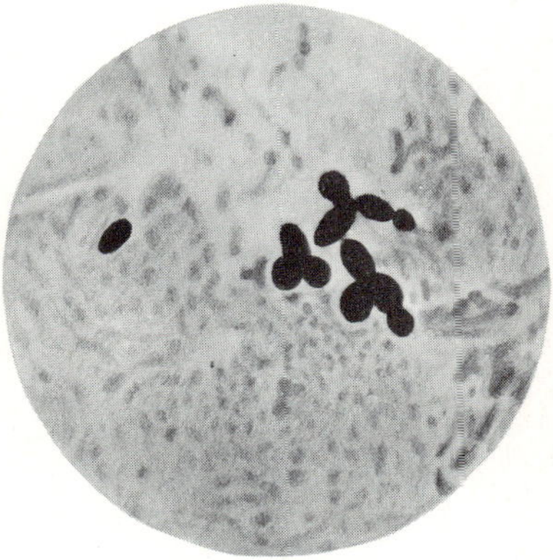

Fig. 30. *Direct vaginal smear from a patient suffering from moniliasis. Note the characteristic dark staining, budding, yeast-like* Candida albicans *(× 1000).*

2. GRAM-NEGATIVE DIVISION

NEISSERIA

Kidney-shaped bodies in pairs, often seen inside pus cells. Found on mucous membranes, particularly upper respiratory tract, genito-urinary tract and conjunctiva.

PATHOGENIC		HARMLESS
N. gonorrhoeae, or gonococcus. Enters through mucous membrane of genito-urinary tract or conjunctiva. Cause of **gonorrhoea** and some cases of **purulent ophthalmia.** Usually seen in direct smears of pus from urethritis and cervicitis	*N. meningitidis,* or meningococcus. Enters through mucous membrane of upper respiratory tract, thence to blood stream and central nervous system. Healthy nasopharyngeal carriers provide the reservoirs of infection. Cause of **cerebrospinal fever.** Also called **meningococcal meningitis.** Found in cerebrospinal fluid in cases of meningitis and usually easily seen in direct smears	*N. catarrhalis, N. pharyngeus,* commensals of the respiratory tract

Both these pathogenic organisms die very quickly outside the body and this must be remembered when material for culture is being taken.

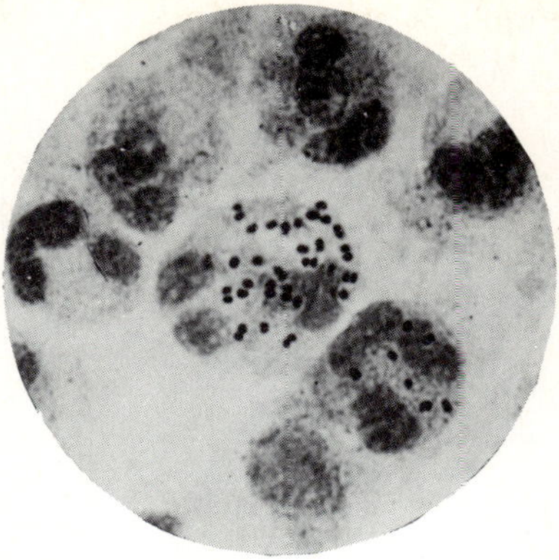

Fig. 31. *Direct smear of urethral discharge from a patient suffering from acute gonorrhoea. Note characteristic intracellular* Neisseria gonorrhoeae *and close similarity to Fig. 32. (× 1000).*

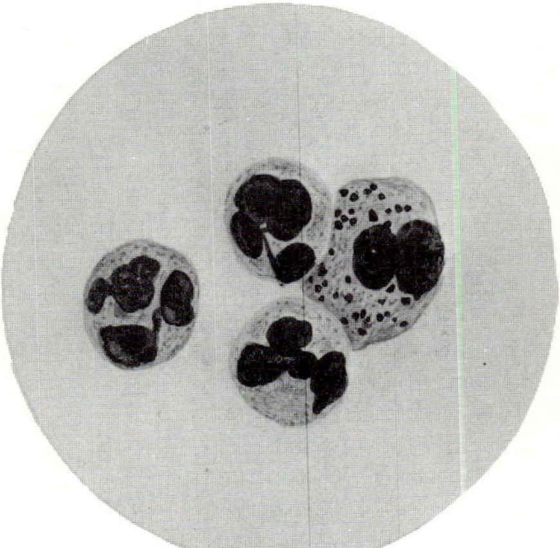

Fig. 32. Smear of cerebrospinal fluid from a case of meningococcal. meningitis. Note pus cells with characteristic intra-cellular Neisseria meningitidis *(× 475).*

HAEMOPHILUS

Very small rod-shaped organisms, but varying greatly in length. Usually inhabit mucous membranes of man and animals.

PATHOGENIC

- *H. ducreyi*. Enters by mucous membrane of genital tract. Cause of **soft sore** or **soft chancre**
- *H. influenzae,** or Pfeiffer's bacillus. Certain strains enter through upper respiratory tract and pass via blood stream into central nervous system. May also infect the conjunctiva. Cause of **meningitis** and **conjunctivitis.** Often found in patients with **chronic bronchitis.**
- *Bordetella pertussis*. Enters by upper respiratory tract. Cause of **whooping cough** or **pertussis**

HARMLESS

- Strains of *H. influenzae* found in the upper respiratory tract of older children and adults.

*Once thought to be the cause of influenza, which we now know is caused by a virus

BRUCELLA

Very small rods. Inhabit animals, particularly cattle, sheep, goats and swine and are excreted in milk of cattle and goats. All the brucellae seem to be pathogenic for man.

Br. suis.	*Br. abortus.*	*Br. melitensis.*
Found in swine. Cause of a type of **undulant fever.** More common in the United States than in Great Britain	Found in cattle. Cause of **undulant fever** or abortus fever. Cause of **abortion in cattle** in Great Britain	Found in goats. Cause of **undulant fever** or Malta fever. Common in Mediterranean countries but not in Great Britain

All the brucellae enter through the mucous membranes of the intestine, either by infected milk or indirectly through personal contact with infected animals. In Great Britain the disease is generally spread through batches of infected milk, though brucellosis is still fairly common in farm hands and veterinary workers. From the intestine the organisms pass into the blood stream, and may be grown from samples of the patient's blood (blood culture). Patients may develop antibodies detectable in serum agglutinin tests, and these tests are carried out on sera of patients with pyrexia of unknown origin.

PASTEURELLA AND ASSOCIATED SPECIES

Small rods with polar granules. Inhabit insects, particularly fleas and ticks, which pass them on to rodents, which in turn infect other insects. Human beings may become involved in the pasteurellae life cycle if brought in contact with certain insects and certain rodents. Some of the pasteurellae are found in animals (e.g. cats) without any known intervention by insects.

P. pestis.
Inhabits the rat flea, which lives on blood of the plague rats. Other fleas bite the infected rats and then bite men, causing **bubonic** or **pneumonic plague**

*P. septica.**
Carried by domestic cats and dogs which transfer the organism by a bite or scratch causing wound infections which are very slow to heal.

* This is not the cause of **cat scratch fever,** which is caused by a virus

In all these infections the organisms usually enter by puncture of the skin, thence via lymphatics to blood stream but they may also be inhaled. This latter is the mode of infection in pneumonic plague.

Francisella tularensis

Inhabits ticks which bite rats and squirrels, which infect other ticks which bite men, causing tularaemia. Unknown in Great Britain, well known in the United States. Tularaemia is generally acquired by persons who handle infected animal carcases.

Yersinia

Infections due to *Yersinia enterocolitica* affecting first animals (e.g. hares, pigs, sheep) and then man, have been spreading rapidly since 1961. The organism is widespread in the environment, in water, and in small mammals which may be healthy carriers. In man, *Yersinia* is a cause of acute enterocolitis. Infection is thought to occur by the faecal–oral route and to be more common in children and adolescents.

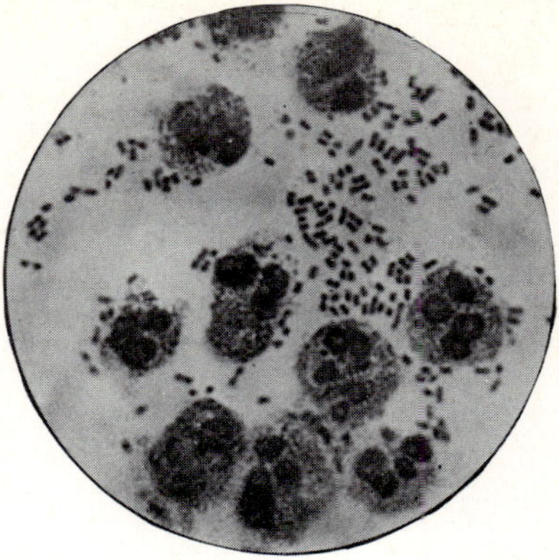

Fig. 33. *Deposit from an infected urine showing pus cells and profuse* Escherichia coli *(× 1000).*

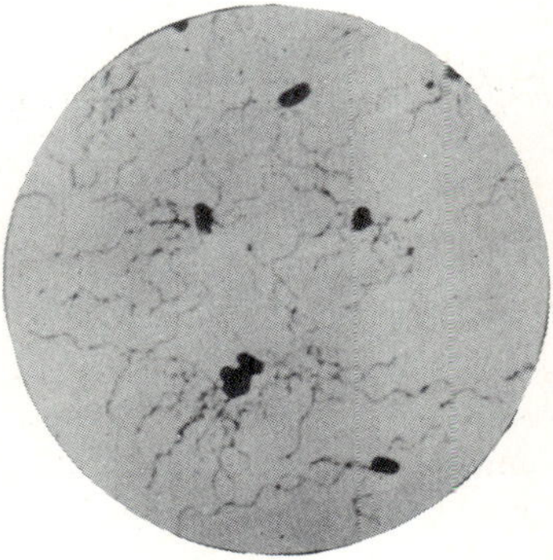

Fig. 34. *Culture smear of* Salmonella typhi *specially stained to show flagellae (× 1500).*

INTESTINAL ORGANISMS

Small rods, sometimes motile, sometimes encapsulated. Widely distributed in nature, in the intestinal tract of man and animals. Some species are pathogenic in the gut; others, e.g the majority of types of *E. coli,* are normal inhabitants of the gut but may be pathogenic elsewhere in the body. Some, such as *Serratia* and *Enterobacter,* are of low pathogenicity. They are sometimes described as opportunists because they are able to take advantage of diminished immune response and to cause superimposed infection in moist, open wounds, or urinary tract infection in association with poor drainage or irrigation equipment.

Escherichia and Klebsiella

These organisms are distinguished from each other by biochemical tests.

Escherichia coli. Found in the urinary tract in pyelitis, pyelonephritis and cystitis. Also found in wounds and may occasionally cause meningitis. Certain types of *E. coli* are associated with neonatal gastroenteritis.

Klebsiella spp. Commonly found in hospital practice causing wound, urinary, respiratory and other infections. Found in relatively small numbers in the normal intestinal tract. *Klebsiella pneumoniae* (Friedlander's bacillus) is found in the respiratory tract and is said to be responsible for about 3% of cases of pneumonia.

Salmonella

Small motile rods, indistinguishable from *Escherichia* except by biochemical and serological tests and inhabiting the same places. All members are pathogenic.

ENTERIC FEVER GROUP

Salmonella typhi (typhoid bacillus) cause of typhoid fever.

Salm. paratyphi B cause of paratyphoid fever in Great Britain.

Salm. paratyphi A common in Asia.

Salm. paratyphi C uncommon in Great Britain, common in Europe.

These organisms enter the intestine in contaminated food, milk or water. They then pass into the lymphatics, thence to the blood stream and bone marrow, and back to the lymphoid tissue of the reticuloendothelial system. They are excreted in faeces, urine, and possibly vomit.

FOOD POISONING GROUP

A large number of named types exist. Commonly found in Great Britain are, e.g. *Salm. typhimurium, Salm. enteriditis, Salm. dublin.* The organisms enter the intestine in food or drink, and they and their effects are confined to the intestinal tract.

Shigella

Small rod, indistinguishable from *Escherichia,* but non-motile. The habitat of these organisms is limited to the intestinal tract of man and other primates.

Sh. shiga.	*Sh. flexneri.*	*Sh. sonnei.*	*Sh. boydii.*
Very rare in Great Britain	6 types fairly common in Great Britain	Very common in Great Britain	Several types, rare in Great Britain

The organisms are the cause of *bacillary dysentery.* They are distinguished from other intestinal organisms by biochemical and serological tests. Infection is spread by human carriers and cases. The organisms produce their effect on the mucous membrane of the large intestine. Besides those mentioned above, *Sh. schmitzi, Sh. alkalescens* and *Sh. dispar* are occasionally found in Great Britain. *Sh. sonnei* is usually found in children, and *Sh. flexneri* is common among patients in mental institutions.

PROTEUS, PSEUDOMONAS AND VIBRIO

Motile rods which are self-sufficient and independent, inhabiting air, soil and especially water, and found in excreta of man and animals.

Proteus spp. There are four species of *Proteus,* but the one most often found in human infections is *P. mirabilis.* This organism commonly infects the urinary tract and its ability to split urea causes the urine to smell of ammonia. It may also be pathogenic in any site outside the intestinal tract.

Pseudomonas aeruginosa (pyocyanea). This organism takes advantage of diminished natural resistance and thus commonly infects, e.g. burns, tracheostomies. It will rapidly colonize wet reservoirs such as humidifiers, sink traps or flower water. It has a characteristic smell and produces a blue/green pigment which may colour pus.

Vibrio. A comma-shaped motile rod. *Vibrio cholera,* the cause of Asiatic cholera, is pathogenic only to man. Infection is spread by water and the organism affects the intestinal tract only. *Vibrio parahaemolyticus* is a cause of food poisoning associated with eating contaminated shellfish. It is particularly common in Japan but occurs elsewhere.

3. BRANCHING BACTERIA AND ACTINOMYCETACEAE

A huge family of organisms which may be Gram-positive, Gram-negative or intermediate. They are distinguished from other bacteria because they branch. They inhabit soil, air, plants and animals and include the streptomyces (source of streptomycin and other antibiotics).

GRAM-POSITIVE MEMBERS

Club-ended Tangled Filaments

Anaerobes

Actinomyces israeli. Method of entry variable. Causes chronic granulomatous lesions of jaw, caecum and appendix, lung etc.

Aerobes

Nocardia madurae. Cause of the tropical disease **Madura foot**

Nocardia asteroides. Causes of **chronic abscess in lungs and muscles**

Rudimentary Branching

Erysipelothrix rhusiopathiae, or swine fever bacillus. Enters through scratch or skin puncture by some article infected by rats or by infected swine. Causes cellulitis of hand and forearm called **erysipeloid** seen often in fish porters. When caught from infected swine there is usually a severe infection

Actinomyces muris, or *Streptobacillus moniliformis.* Enters through skin by rat bite or scratch, but may be taken in infected milk. Causes fever, rash, endocarditis and polyarthritis, which is sometimes called **Haverhill fever** or **rat-bite fever**

GRAM-NEGATIVE MEMBERS

Bacteroides spp. A large group of non-sporing anaerobic, usually Gram-negative, bacteria. Normal inhabitants of genital and intestinal tracts, but they may cause severe postoperative wound infections, often in association with other organisms, e.g. peritonitis following bowel surgery. *Bacteroides* spp. are the most numerous of the gut commensals.

Fusiform spp. (fusiform bacilli). Fusiform bacilli accompanied by *Borrelia vincentii* (p. 136) are found in smears of mouth, gums and fauces in the ulcerative gingivitis known as *Vincent's angina*.

Mycoplasma. Characterized by absence of cell wall and therefore of indefinite shapes and sizes. Aerobic, difficult to grow. Group also known as PPLO (pleuro-pneumonia-like organisms), so called because they resemble the organisms which cause pleuro-pneumonia in cattle. Found on mucous membranes of eyes and genitalia.

Mycoplasma pneumoniae causes primary atypical pneumonia.

4. ACID-FAST DIVISION

MYCOBACTERIUM

Slender rods, are enveloped with unsaponifiable wax which renders the organisms difficult to stain by Gram's method. After staining by hot carbol fuchsin, the organisms are stain-fast, resisting decolorization with alcohols and strong mineral acids. Non-pathogenic forms are widely distributed in nature, e.g. *Myco. smegmatis, Myco. butyricum.*

PATHOGENIC

- *Myco. leprae.* Cannot be cultured and is not pathogenic for animals. Cause of **leprosy** which is diagnosed microscopically from scrapings or sections of material from patients
- *Myco. tuberculosis,* or tubercle bacilli
  - Human type; cause of **pulmonary tuberculosis**
  - Bovine type; cause of **body and glandular tuberculosis**
- A number of strains of low pathogenicity, e.g. *Myco. balnei* cause of **swimming pool granuloma**

Mycobacterium tuberculosis is a slow growing organism. If present in sufficiently large numbers it may be seen on direct microscopy but before a laboratory diagnosis of tuberculosis can be confirmed or eliminated it has to be grown on a special culture medium. This may take as long as six to eight weeks.

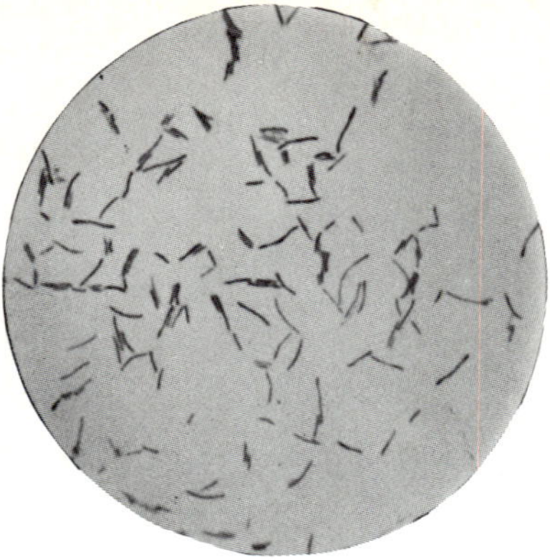

Fig. 35. *Culture smear of* Mycobacterium tuberculosis *(× 1500). Note characteristic slightly curved, delicate bacilli.*

5. SPIROCHAETES

Slender rods, moving by flexing and corkscrew motion. Visualized by dark ground illumination of the microscope field because they are difficult or impossible to stain by usual methods. Non-pathogenic spirochaetes are found in the mouth, on gums and the genitalia.

PATHOGENIC

Leptospira. Corkscrew-shaped with hooked ends

Many species, e.g. *L. icterohaemorrhagiae.* Cause of **infectious jaundice or Weil's disease.** Carried by rats and enters through contamination of damaged skin or mucous membrane, associated with sewer workers

Treponema. Very delicate regular coils

Trep. pallidum Cause of **syphilis.** Enters through mucous membrane of genito-urinary tract, mouth, or other direct contact site

Trep. pertenue. Cause of **yaws,** in tropical countries. Spread by direct contact with skin lesions

Borrelia. Large, wormlike

Borrelia recurrentis and *Borrelia duttoni* are carried by lice or ticks to human hosts who develop **relapsing fever** (tropical countries). *Borrelia vincentii* (or Vincent's spirochaete) accompanied by *Fusiformis* sp. are found in the ulcerative condition of the mouth and gums known as **Vincent's angina**

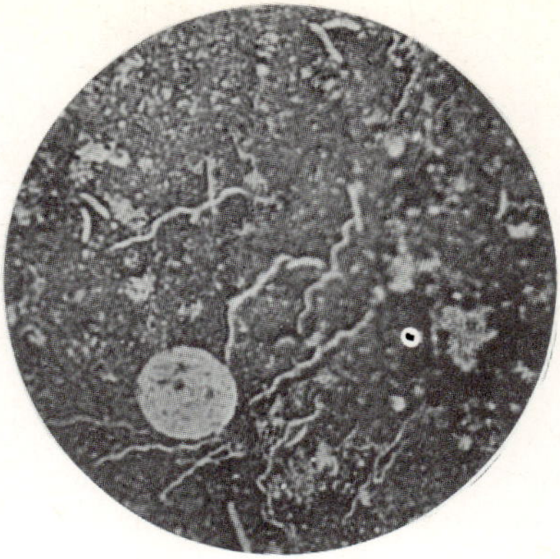

Fig. 36. *Direct smear from the throat of a patient with Vincent's angina. Note the characteristic spirochaetes and fusiform bacilli (×1000).*

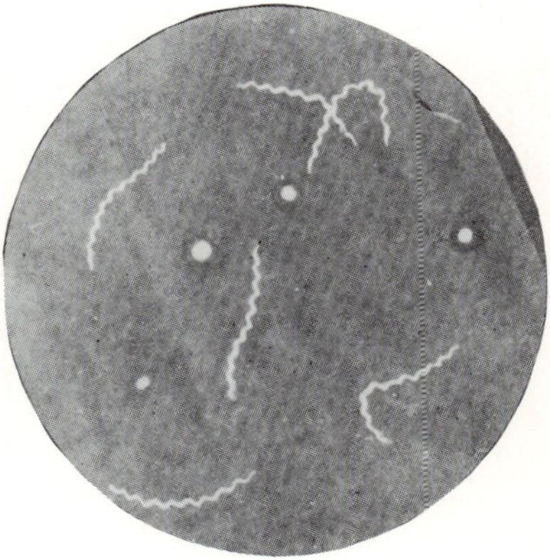

Fig. 37. Treponema pallidum *from a primary syphilitic lesion (× 1000).*

6. RICKETTSIAE

Rickettsiae are grouped between bacteria and viruses. Specimens are tested for Rickettsiae in the virology laboratory (see page 166).

R. prowazeki. Cause of **epidemic typhus,** is transmitted by lice	*R. orientalis.* Cause of **scrub typhus,** is transmitted by mites	*R. rickettsi.* Cause of **spotted fever,** is transmitted by ticks

Each of the different forms of typhus and spotted fever is caused by different rickettsiae, which are carried by insects indigenous to the places where they occur, e.g. Rocky Mountain spotted fever, South African tick-bite fever, Queensland tick-bite fever. Q fever caused by *R. burnetii* has occurred in Britain since the Second World War.

7. VIRUSES

The many varieties of virus and the diseases that they cause are outlined in Chapter 10.

Summary of Bacterial Transmission

Pathogen	*Portal of Entry*	*Clinical Disease*	*Route of Exit*	*Usual Source of Infection*	*Accommodation*
Streptococcus (beta haemolytic streptococcus Group A)	Upper respiratory tract	Tonsillitis	Respiratory secretions	Human cases and throat and nasal carriers	Single room for 48 hours
		Otitis media	Aural and respiratory secretions		Systemic penicillin then ward if apyrexial
		Meningitis	None		
		Secondary pneumonia	Sputum		
	Any route, usually upper respiratory tract	Scarlet fever	Secretions from lesions and respiratory		
	Skin	Erysipelas, cellulitis			
		Wound infection	Pus from lesions		
	Locally at placental site	Puerperal sepsis	Lochia		
	Possible sequelae to listed infections	Rheumatic fever	None		Ward
		Acute nephritis	None		Ward
Streptococcus pneumoniae (pneumococcus)	Respiratory tract	Pneumonia	Sputum	Commensal organism, opportunist, i.e. infection only when contributory factor, e.g. damaged mucosa, congestion	Ward
		Sinusitis	Nasal secretions		
		Otitis media	Aural and respiratory nasal secretions		
	Middle ear, sinuses	Meningitis	None		Ward
	Conjunctiva	Conjunctivitis	Conjunctival secretions		Ward
Streptococcus faecalis	Gut lesions to blood stream	Subacute bacterial endocarditis	None	Gut	Ward
	Contact transmission	Wound infection	Pus from lesions		Ward

Pathogen	*Portal of Entry*	*Clinical Disease*	*Route of Exit*	*Usual Source of Infection*	*Accommodation*
Streptococcus faecalis	Via urethra	Urinary tract infection	Urine		Ward
Staphylococcus aureus (*Staphylococcus pyogenes*, coagulase positive *Staphylococcus*)	Local, skin	Boils, carbuncles, whitlows, impetigo, wound infections	Pus from lesions	Human cases and carriers Transmission by hands, equipment, bedding and clothing	Single room unless very minor lesion
	Surgery	Deep abscesses	Pus after incision		
	Blood stream	Osteomyelitis	Pus after incision		
	Respiratory tract	Otitis media	Discharge from ear		
		Pneumonia	Sputum		
	Ingestion of infected food, carbo-hydrate, e.g. trifle, custard	Toxic vomiting (food poisoning)	Faeces and vomit for a few hours. N.B. any remaining food dangerous	Enterotoxin strain in staff handling food, e.g. septic finger	Ward
	From skin or deep infection	Septicaemia	None (excluding initial lesion)		
Neisseria gonorrhoeae (*gonococcus*)	Direct spread during coitus	Gonorrhoea ♂ Urethritis, epidi-dymitis, prostatis ♀ Urethritis, cervici-tis, vulvovaginitis, salpingitis	Discharges from urethra and vagina	Human cases	Single room for 48 hours; systemic penicillin then ward
	Blood stream from primary	Arthritis	None		Ward
	Eye	Ophthalmia neonatorum	Conjunctival secretions	Maternal vaginal discharge	Single room

Neisseria meningitidis (meningococcus)	Respiratory tract	Meningitis (cerebro-spinal fever)	Nasal secretions	Human nasopharyngeal carriers, close contact transmission	Single room until nasopharyngeal secretions negative (usually 48 hours) then ward
		Septicaemia with rash and arthritis	Skin lesions		
	Eye	Ophthalmitis	Discharge from eyes		
Corynebacterium diphtheriae	Respiratory tract	Diphtheria Organism infects nasal cavity, pharynx, tonsils, larynx, trachea; rarely conjunctiva, wound or vagina: toxin absorbed from these sites cause the disease	Respiratory tract secretions	Cases, convalescent cases, and carriers (usually in nose or throat)	Isolation unit until 2 negative nasal and 2 negative throat swabs
	Local		From secretions		Usually up to 14 days
Mycobacterium tuberculosis (tubercle bacillus)	Respiratory tract Ingestion	Tuberculosis (*a*) Pulmonary (*b*) Cervical glands (*c*) Alimentary tract	Sputum Discharging sinus Faeces	Open cases Infected milk Infected or swallowed sputum	(*a*) Tuberculosis unit or single room until negative culture (*b*) and (*c*) Preferably single room
	Lymphatic/blood stream spread of primary	Miliary tuberculosis Meningitis Bone + joint lesions	Any open lesion		
		Kidney lesions	Urine		
		Testicular lesions Fallopian tube plus uterine lesions	Menstrual fluid		
Mycobacterium leprae	Direct contact, probably through skin or mucous membrane	Leprosy (*a*) Cutaneous (nodular) (*b*) Neural (anaesthetic)	Skin lesions	Close, continuous contact with an open case, e.g. familial	Ward

Pathogen	Portal of Entry	Clinical Disease	Route of Exit	Usual Source of Infection	Accommodation
Bacillus anthracis	 Direct contact Inhalation of spores	Anthrax (*a*) Cutaneous (*b*) Pulmonary (wool sorters' disease)	 Skin lesions Sputum	Infected animal hides and furs, etc.	Isolation unit. Rarely transmitted man to man, spore contaminated items may remain infective for years
Clostridium tetani	Injury, usually a puncture wound	Tetanus Symptoms due to powerful neuro-toxin	Discharging wound	Soil containing spores from animal faeces	Usually non-infective. Single room required for other medical reasons
Clostridium welchii (perfringens) and related strains	Contamination of devitalized muscle	Gas gangrene Symptoms due to toxaemia, may lead to septicaemia	Discharge from lesion	Present in faeces of normal man and animals	Hyperbaric O_2 unit Ward
Heat resistant Type A strains	Ingestion	Food poisoning diarrhoea		Contaminated food	Ward
Clostridium botulinum	Ingestion	Botulism. A pure toxaemia, about 70% mortality	None. Organism grows in food, not in intestine	Rare. Home canned vegetables or home cured meat	Ward Assisted respiration
Actinomyces israeli	Ingestion	Actinomycosis Subacute or chronic granulomatous disease Suppuration and fistulae, usually cervicofacial, abdominal or thoracic	Discharge from lesions	Endogenous. Normal mouth flora, opportunist organism	Ward

Treponema pallidum	(*a*) Placenta	Congenital syphilis	Secretions of respiratory tract (nasal + lung lesion)	Syphylitic mother	Single room for 48 hrs Systemic penicillin then ward
	(*b*) Skin or mucous membrane	Primary syphilis (chancre)	Discharge from chancre	Direct contact during coitus	
	Via blood stream	Secondary syphilis	Discharge from surface lesions e.g. mouth ulcer	Contact with infected lesions, e.g. coitus, kissing, mouth care	Ward
		Tertiary syphilis Gummata, dementia, meningo and cardiovascular tabes	None other than discharge from surface gumma		
Leptospira icterohaemorrhagiae	Ingestion, or by abrasions in skin or mucous membrane	Weil's disease (spirochaetal jaundice). Common in sewer workers	Urine	Rats spread organism and excrete it in urine. Contaminated water	Ward
Borrelia vincentii	Mouth normal flora, opportunist organism	Vincent's angina, with a fusiform bacillus	Respiratory secretions	Human carriers or cases	Ward
Escherichia coli	Via urethra	Urinary tract infection	Urine	Gut and faecal contamination	Ward
	Perforated gut	Peritonitis	None		
	Contact transmission	Infection of wounds, burns	Discharge from lesions		
Enteropathogenic strains	Ingestion	Diarrhoea in infants and the very old	Faeces	Human carriers or cases	Isolation unit

Pathogen	*Portal of Entry*	*Clinical Disease*	*Route of Exit*	*Usual Source of Infection*	*Accommodation*
Salmonella Enteric fever group: *S. typhi, S. paratyphi*	Ingestion	Enteric fever (typhoid and paratyphoid)	All secretions during septicaemia for first two weeks: faeces, urine	Human carriers or cases via water or food	Single room
Food poisoning group: *Salmonella typhimurium* and over 800 others		Gastroenteritis	Vomit and faeces	Human or animal carriers or cases via food	
Shigella, numerous types, e.g. *sonnei*	Ingestion	Bacillary dysentery	Faeces	Human carriers or cases	Single room
Proteus mirabilis	Via urethra	Urinary tract infection	Urine	Gut, nasal, external ear carriers	Depends on the extent and severity of the infection
	Contact transmission	Wound and respiratory infections	Discharges		
Pseudomonas aeruginosa (Pseudomonas pyocyanea)	Contact transmission	Infection in tissues damaged by disease, accident or surgery, e.g. bronchiectasis, burns, tracheostomy, surgical wound and urinary tract infection	Secretions and discharges	Organism often present in the gut Reservoirs in wet situations, e.g. humidifiers, sink traps, flower water etc.	Depends on the extent and severity of the infection
Klebsiella spp.	Some strains normally present in respiratory tract	Respiratory tract infections, e.g. pneumonia	Nasal and bronchial secretions	Endogenous. Easily transmissible via wet media, hands, instruments	Depends on the extent and severity of the infection

	Contact transmission	Wound infections	Discharges		
	Via urethra	Urinary tract infection	Urine		
Vibrio cholera	Ingestion	Asiatic cholera Diarrhoea and vomiting Affects intestinal tract only	Faeces and vomit	Human cases or carriers via contaminated water or food	Isolation unit
Haemophilus influenzae	Respiratory tract	Secondary respiratory tract infections; infects mucosa damaged by influenza virus	Respiratory secretions	Often found as normal mouth flora, some cause infection	Ward
		Meningitis in children	None		
		Septic arthritis	None		
	Conjunctiva	Conjunctivitis	Conjunctival secretions		
Haemophilus ducreyi	Direct contact during coitus	Soft chancre (chancroid)	Discharge from chancre	Human case, intercourse	
Bordetella pertussis	Respiratory tract	Whooping cough	Respiratory secretions	Cases	Isolation unit
Brucella abortus *Brucella melitensis*	Ingestion	Brucellosis (undulant and Malta fevers)	Usually none, occasionally in urine	Unpasteurized cow's or goat's milk	Ward
Candida albicans (Monilia)	Damaged tissues	Candidiasis: Mouth (thrush) Skin, septic fingers Vagina Systemic	Exudates	Often found in normal mouth, vagina, intestines Opportunist organism	Ward except for very severe infection, then single room

10 A Guide to Common Viruses

There are three important ways in which viruses differ from other micro-organisms:

1. They are so small that many of them are not visible with a light microscope, though they can be studied with an electron microscope. Viruses vary in size from about 20 to 300 nm whereas staphylococci measure 1000 nm.
2. They possess either DNA or RNA, but never both types of nucleic acid (p. 14).
3. Neither viruses nor rickettsiae can grow on lifeless media, but only within living susceptible cells.

Structure

Virus particles consist of a core of nucleic acid (DNA or RNA) surrounded by a protein coat (capsid). Some viruses, e.g. herpesvirus, are enclosed by a further layer or envelope. The capsid protects the nucleic acid and facilitates the attachment of the virus to the host cell, it also contains antigenic material which is specific for each virus type. Electron microscopy studies have demonstrated three types of virus symmetry; cubic, helical and complex. The nucleocapsid of a virus with cubic symmetry is usually icosahedral, i.e. contained by twenty plane faces, e.g. adenovirus. The nucleocapsid of a virus with helical symmetry is elongated and wound in the form of a helix or spiral, e.g. influenza. Those which are neither cubic nor helical are described as having complex symmetry, e.g. smallpox.

Infection

Many infections are known to be due to viruses; others are believed to be when no bacterial source of infection can be demonstrated in an obviously transmissible disease. Virus infections are common and most are mild (e.g. colds). Some are called 'silent' and commonly multiply in the body without causing disease (e.g. cytomegalovirus), some cause latent infection (e.g. herpes simplex), a few cause very severe or fatal illness (e.g. smallpox).

Many viruses enter the body by inhalation (e.g. influenza, measles), others gain entry by ingestion (e.g. poliomyelitis), or inoculation (e.g. hepatitis B), all spread locally directly to the tissues and some are disseminated widely via the blood stream. Viruses invade living cells and 'take over' the cell metabolic processes to reproduce themselves; the cell usually dies and releases the virus particles but it may survive and carry the virus as in latent infections. Certain viruses can induce changes in the genetic material of cells causing them to undergo malignant transformation.

Defence Mechanisms

Cells invaded and infected by a virus produce a protein substance, *interferon,* in the acute stage of the disease. This is released and temporarily protects other cells which take it up, from infection. Viral antigens stimulate the production of antibodies which are carried in the patient's serum and neutralize any subsequent invasion by the same virus, i.e. the patient becomes immune to that virus. Specific immunity, of which circulating antibody is one manifestation, persists often for many years, but may gradually decrease to a level where the patient is again susceptible or partially susceptible to infection. For example, herpes zoster (shingles) occurring in an adult is due to the same virus which caused his childhood attack of varicella (chickenpox); the second infection occurs when the immunity level has decreased.

Destruction of Viruses

Most viruses are killed by exposure to heat such as boiling for a few minutes, but survive storage at temperatures as low as −70°C. Their ability to withstand drying is very variable but all are thought to be sensitive to ultra-violet light. In general terms viruses can be destroyed by the action of aldehydes, chlorine, iodine and hydrogen peroxide; some are completely resistant to the phenolic group of disinfectants; a chlorine derivative, e.g. Chloros, hypochlorite, is commonly used for disinfection purposes. The advice of a virologist should be taken in outbreaks of infection since different viruses vary in their reaction to chemicals.

Only certain viruses contain lipid and the fact that lipid-containing viruses are inactivated by ether or chloroform is used in the laboratory identification and classification of viruses.

Laboratory Identification

Light microscopy. Particles of 300 nm can be resolved. Inclusion bodies may be present in tissue cells as a result of virus infection. They are seen as clumps of virus particles within the cytoplasm, e.g. trachoma, or as an eosinophilic mass in the cell nucleus, e.g. herpes.

Electron microscopy. Using a beam of electrons focussed by magnets structures as small as 0·5 nm can be resolved.

Antibody titre. Two blood samples are compared. The first is taken in the acute phase of illness, the second about 14 days later. Recent infection is indicated by a significant rise in titre or, less satisfactorily, by a high level of antibodies to the infecting virus in both samples or a late convalescent sample when no earlier sample is available.

Culture. Viruses can be grown in the laboratory by inoculating:

1. A tissue culture of cells grown in a single layer on the wall of a glass test tube.
2. Chick embryo in fertile hens' eggs.
3. Laboratory animals.

Classification

Classification of viruses is at a relatively early stage. At the present time they are grouped according to their nucleic acid composition, size and symmetry, structure, sensitivity to ether, and by the diseases which they cause.

ADENOVIRUS GROUP

DNA viruses. Icosahedral. 75 nm.

Diagnostic material: Mouth washings, throat swabs, faeces, conjunctival swabs (in eye disease).

There are 31 serotypes in this group; the viruses attack lymphoid tissue and may cause:

Pharyngitis	Conjunctivitis	Mesenteric adenitis
	May be spread by eye instruments	

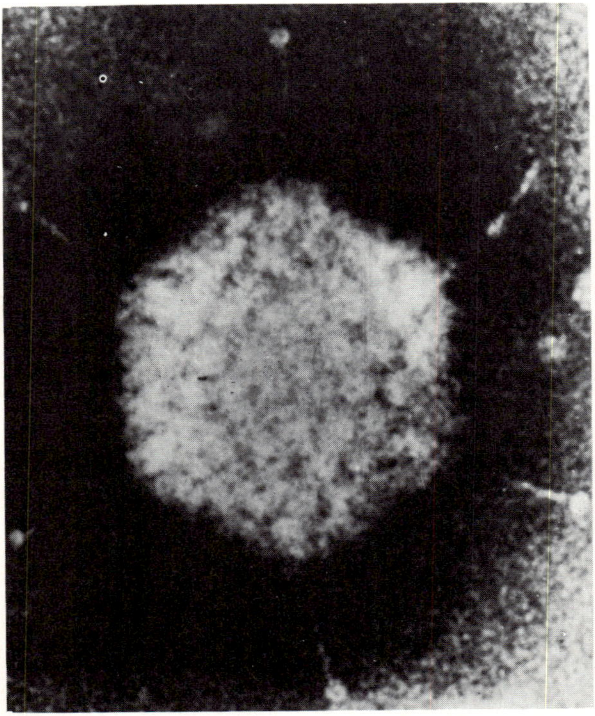

Fig. 38. *An adenovirus as seen through the electron microscope.*

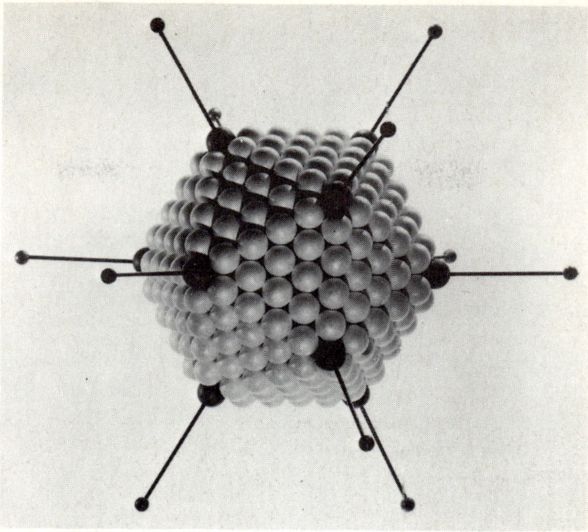

Fig. 39. *Model of adenovirus showing its 'antennae'.*

HERPESVIRUS GROUP

DNA viruses. Icosahedral with an outer envelope. 120–200 nm.

Diagnostic material: Vesicle fluid, skin swabs, saliva, conjuctival fluid/scrapings (eye cases); urine (*cytomegalovirus*); cervical, vaginal swabs (herpes genitalis)

Chemotherapy: Cytosine arabinoside. Idoxuridine is of limited value.

These viruses are common in man, often causing symptomless and latent infections, e.g. most adults have antibodies to both herpes simplex and cytomegalovirus without symptoms or history of infection.

Herpes simplex. Primary infection in early childhood is often mild or unrecognized, but may cause gingivostomatitis or conjunctivitis. Other primary infections are *herpes genitalis,* i.e. *Herpesvirus hominis* Type II (venereal transmission), whitlow from contact during nursing care, encephalitis, severe generalized neonatal infection which may be acquired at birth. 'Cold sores' are common recurrent episodes of infection, the virus is thought to remain latent in the trigeminal nerve ganglion between attacks and to be reactivated by non-specific stimuli, e.g. sun, colds. Recurrent infection of the eye causes dendritic corneal ulcers.

Varicella/zoster. *Varicella* (chickenpox) is the primary infection. The virus then remains latent in nerve ganglia; when the level of immunity decreases it may be reactivated, resulting in an attack of *zoster* (shingles). Zoster is not usually acquired by contact with another case or with varicella, but it may cause varicella in susceptible persons, e.g. a nurse who has not had chickenpox. Patients undergoing immunosuppressive therapy are particularly susceptible to varicella/zoster.

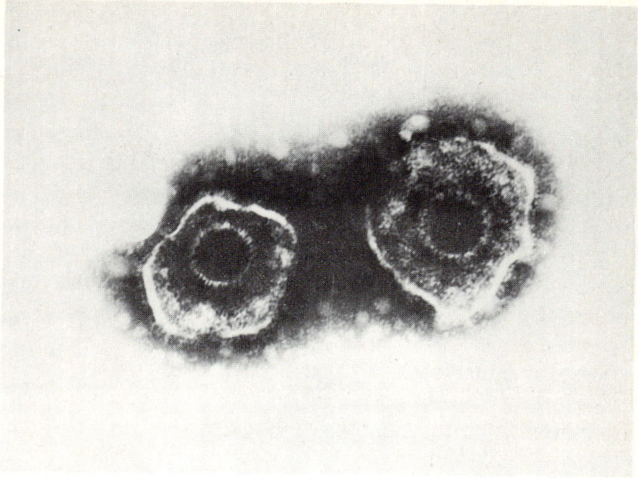

Fig. 40. *Herpesvirus from a vesicle of a patient suffering from chickenpox (× 84 000).*

Cytomegalovirus. Commonly symptomless, but it may cause severe generalized neonatal infection, hepatitis in children or an illness similar to glandular fever in adults. Widespread infection may occur when immunity is impaired.

Epstein-Barr virus. This virus causes infectious mononucleosis (glandular fever). It has also been found to be associated with Burkitt's lymphoma though it is uncertain whether it actually causes this tumour.

POXVIRUS GROUP

DNA viruses. Brick-shaped, complex structure. 200–300 nm.

Diagnostic material: Vesicle fluid, crusts, scrapings from maculo-papules

This virus group includes:

Variola (smallpox)	**Variola minor** (alastrim)	**Vaccinia** Used for smallpox vaccine	Many animal pox viruses

Variola (smallpox) is a severe disease with a high mortality rate in unvaccinated persons. Smallpox vaccine is prepared from closely related, but less virulent, vaccinia virus. Complete immunity last for about three years after vaccination but partial protection which modifies the severity of the disease lasts for considerably longer. A valid international certificate of vaccination (vaccination or revaccination within three years) is required for entry to the United Kingdom from travellers who within the preceding 14 days have been in a country, any part of which is infected (January 1976). When a case of smallpox is detected the patient is nursed in strict isolation and every effort made to trace all contacts immediately; vaccine has to be given early in the incubation period, which averages 12 days, to be effective. Patients with smallpox are strictly isolated, usually in a special unit, because although the main route of infection is by respiratory spread, the virus can survive for years in disseminated, dried skin scabs.

The WHO smallpox eradication programme reported the last known case of variola major in Bangladesh in October 1975. Surveillance will be maintained. Although alastrim, a milder form, is known to persist in Ethiopia it is hoped that variola major has been eradicated world wide.

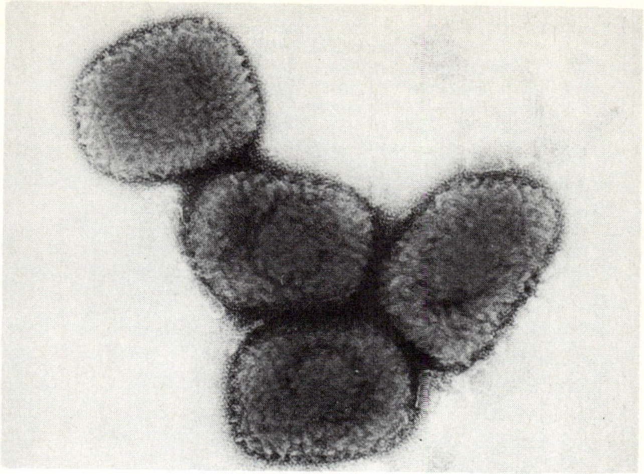

Fig. 41. *Smallpox virus (× 84 000).*

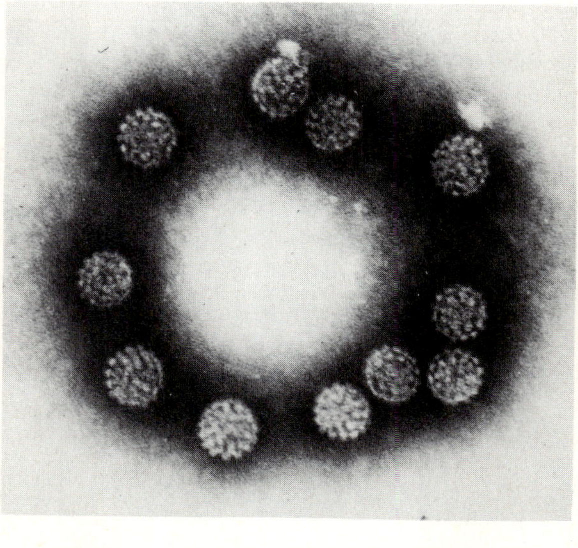

Fig. 42. *Wart virus (× 150 000) from a plantar wart.*

MYXOVIRUS GROUP

RNA viruses. Helical. 80–100 nm

Diagnostic material: Mouth washings, throat swabs.

Influenza A virus is the principal cause of epidemic influenza.

Influenza B virus causes smaller epidemics and outbreaks.

Both viruses attack and desquamate the epithelium of the respiratory tract leaving it susceptible to secondary bacterial invasion, e.g. staphylococcal infection.

Influenza C virus rarely causes clinical infection.

Influenza virus vaccines are available, they give some protection but are not always effective because of the multiplicity of strains. The viruses, particularly influenza A, develop variant strains. Occasionally completely new strains emerge to which the whole world population is susceptible; a pandemic then occurs. Influenza spreads very rapidly, the incubation period is short (two days) and the speed of spread of a new strain often makes it impossible to prepare enough vaccine in time to protect everybody. It is usual therefore to restrict protection to, for example, people with chronic respiratory disease and essential hospital and public service staff. Vaccine must be given before an epidemic starts since antibiodies are not formed instantaneously.

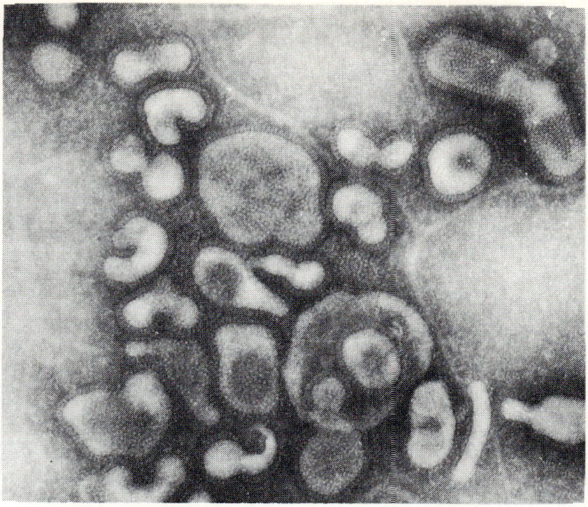

Fig. 43. *Influenza virus (× 75 000) grown in fertile eggs for vaccine production.*

PARAMYXOVIRUS GROUP

RNA viruses. Helical. 90–250 nm

Diagnostic material: Mouth washings, nasal secretions, throat swabs (parainfluenza)

Parotitis (mumps)	**Measles**	**Parainfluenzae** Croup < 5 years	**Respiratory syncytial virus** (RSV) Bronchiolitis in young children

Measles. In the United Kingdom and other countries where living conditions are good the disease is usually mild, but in countries where nutrition levels and living conditions are poor, measles is a serious disease and frequently fatal. In the United Kingdom immunization is given in childhood to avoid the complications, e.g. respiratory tract infections, encephalitis, which occur in some cases. When a child develops measles after admission to a nursery or hospital ward it is usual to protect susceptible contacts by administering

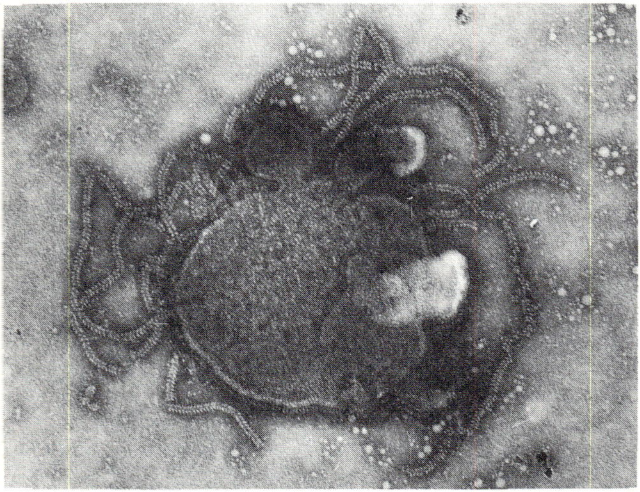

Fig. 44. *Mumps virus (× 50 000).*

gamma-globulin. Gamma-globulin is prepared from pooled human serum (i.e. from many donors) which contains antibody to measles because most adults have had the disease. This is an example of passive immunization.

RUBELLA VIRUS

RNA virus. About 60 nm
Diagnostic material: Blood

Rubella (German measles) is a mild illness but if the disease is transmitted to a pregnant woman during the first four months of pregnancy the virus may cause congenital defects in the fetus, e.g. deafness, cataract, heart defects. In the United Kingdom rubella virus vaccine is given to 12–13-year-old girls, it may also be offered to women in whom the haemagglutination inhibition test is negative (who have not had the disease), but in this case it is important that pregnancy is avoided for two months after vaccination to ensure that there is no possibility of fetal infection due to the attenuated virus. The aim is to protect against rubella before childbearing age without attempting to prevent cases in children.

CORONAVIRUS GROUP

RNA viruses. 100 nm

Little is as yet known about these viruses other than that they can cause respiratory disease.

VIRAL HEPATITIS

Hepatitis A: RNA virus. 28 nm
Hepatitis B: DNA virus. 42 nm
Diagnostic material: Blood

Virus A (*infectious hepatitis*) is transmitted from person to person by faecally contaminated water or food. The disease is endemic in most countries and has an incubation period of 15–50 days, it spreads easily in close contact situations, e.g. families, schools. No active immunization is available against infectious hepatitis but human immunoglobulin is given for short-term passive immunity (3–6 months).

Virus B *(serum hepatitis)* is transmitted from person to person by inoculation of infected blood e.g. from a contaminated hypodermic syringe and needle, medical and laboratory equipment, tattooing. It is also venereally transmitted.

The incubation period of hepatitis B is 50 to 150 days and the disease is differentiated from hepatitis A by testing for antigen in the blood serum. Hepatitis B antigen (Australia antigen or HBs Ag) can be detected only in the serum of patients who are incubating, or actually have hepatitis B, or in jaundice-free persons who still carry the antigen from a previous episode. The silent carriage rate amongst the indigenous population in Great Britain is about 1 in 1000. It is known to be greater in high risk groups, e.g. drug addicts or patients in renal dialysis units, and in some overseas populations, e.g. in Africa and Mediterranean countries.

A limited quantity of specific human immunoglobulin is now available. This gives passive immunity and may be administered following accidental inoculation of infected blood.

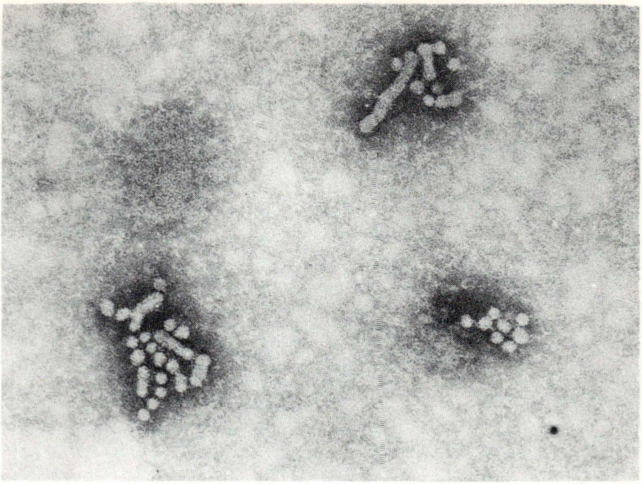

Fig. 45. *Australia antigen (×84 000) from the serum of a patient suffering from serum hepatitis.*

PICORNAVIRUS GROUP

RNA viruses. Small icosahedral. 26 nm
Diagnostic material: Faeces, throat swabs, cerebrospinal fluid (*ECHO virus*), nasal secretions, mouth washings (*Rhinovirus*)

Rhinoviruses. 50 serotypes. Main cause of common colds.

Enteroviruses. Poliovirus, ECHO virus, Coxsackie virus, are ingested, multiply in the alimentary tract and spread from the gut to tissues and organs via the blood stream. Virus is excreted in the faeces.

Poliovirus causes poliomyelitis, but symptomless infection with intestinal carriage is common. There are three serological types of poliovirus; attenuated strains of each type are incorporated in trivalent oral poliovaccine. Immunization with poliovaccine should be given in childhood (p. 42), but the vaccine should also be given to adults such as hospital staff who have not previously been immunized, and may be exposed to the virus.

Coxsackie viruses cause 'hand, foot and mouth' disease, herpangina, Bornholm disease (epidemic myalgia), myocarditis and pericarditis.

Many of the enteroviruses can cause aseptic meningitis and all are common where living conditions and hygiene are poor, though most infections are symptomless.

REOVIRUS GROUP

RNA virus. 60–66 nm. Icosahedral
Diagnostic material: Faeces

Rotavirus, so called (T. H. Flewett 1974) because it looks like a wheel, has recently been identified in outbreaks of gastroenteritis and febrile diarrhoea in infants and young children. Infection occurs most commonly during the winter months and in children under

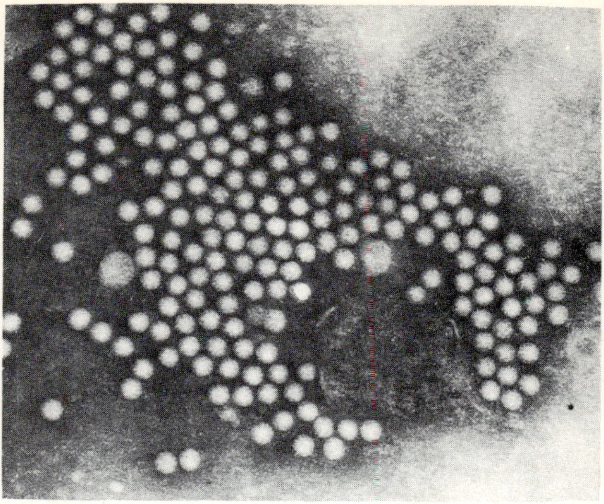

Fig. 46. *Poliovirus (× 100 000). Particles from a purified vaccine.*

three years old. The virus is transmissible by the faecal–oral route and usually causes only mild to moderately severe disease.

ARBOVIRUS GROUP

RNA viruses. 20–150 nm
Diagnostic material: Blood
Important diseases caused include:

Yellow fever	**Encephalitis**	**Systemic febrile disease**

About 50 serotypes cause disease in man. The hosts are birds and small mammals and the virus is transmitted to man by the bite of infected arthropods, i.e. mosquito, tick, sandfly. The diseases are common in many parts of the world though not in the United Kingdom. Yellow fever virus vaccine should preferably not be given at the same time as smallpox or poliovirus vaccines.

ARENOVIRUS GROUP

RNA viruses. 70–150 nm
Diagnostic material: Blood, throat washings

Lassa fever is an acute infectious disease first recognized in West Africa in 1969. In endemic areas the virus is transmitted to man in food contaminated by the urine or saliva of an infected rat (*Mastomys natalensis*). Person-to-person transmission is by close contact with the blood, pharyngeal secretions or urine of an infected patient.

Modern air travel increases the risk of tropical fevers such as Lassa fever and Marburg disease reaching this country. Patients are nursed in strict isolation and only in scheduled units because to date there is no specific treatment or vaccine available.

RHABDOVIRUS GROUP

RNA viruses. Bullet-shaped, helical. 37–60 nm
Diagnostic material: Saliva, cerebrospinal fluid, urine

Rabies virus is transmitted from infected dogs, cats, bats, or carnivorous wild animals in the saliva, by biting. The virus spreads from the wound to the central nervous system via nerve tissue and the disease is fatal. The long incubation period (usually 4–12 weeks) makes prophylactic active immunization after exposure possible. A combination of anti-rabies vaccine (active immunization) and heterologous anti-rabies serum or human anti-rabies immunoglobulin (passive immunization) is usually given.

RICKETTSIAE

Rickettsiae are grouped between viruses and bacteria. Like viruses they multiply only within living cells, but like bacteria contain both RNA and DNA. They can be visualized with a light microscope although slightly smaller than bacteria.

The group includes:

R. prowazeki	*R. mooseri*	*R. orientalis*	*R. rickettsi*	*C. burneti*
Typhus fever	Murine typhus	Tsutsuga-mushi fever	Rocky mountain spotted fever	Q fever
Louse-borne	Flea-borne	Mite-borne	Tick-borne	

Epidemic typhus fever is associated with very poor, overcrowded living conditions and is transmitted by the victim scratching infected louse faeces into the skin. It is an epidemic disease, control measures are directed towards eliminating lice; vaccine is available.

Q fever is primarily a disease of large domestic animals, transmitted to man in the milk of infected cows or sheep and by inhalation of dust contaminated by placentae, fetal membranes and fluid after the birth of a calf to an infected animal. The patient may have atypical pneumonia, pyrexia, or a subacute endocarditis if the heart valves are already damaged.

CHLAMYDIAE

Chlamydiae are grouped between viruses and bacteria. They multiply only within living cells as do viruses, but like bacteria contain both RNA and DNA, can be visualized with a light microscope and measure 250–450 nm.

Psittacosis (ornithosis)	**Lympho-granuloma venereum**	**TRIC agents**	**Non-specific urethritis and cervicitis**

TRIC (trachoma–inclusion conjunctivitis agents) are widespread in tropical countries and associated with poor living conditions and lack of hygiene. The agent is spread by contact, contaminated communal possessions and flies, and is a common cause of blindness. In temperate climates they cause non-specific urethritis and cervicitis or conjunctivitis.

Summary of Viral Transmission

Virus	*Entry Route*	*Disease*	*Exit Route*	*Usual Source of Infection*	*Accommodation*
Pox group					
Variola Variola minor	Inhalation	Smallpox	Respiratory secretions vesicle fluid. Dried scabs may remain infectious for years	Cases	Isolation unit until scabs have gone. Average 2–3 weeks
Vaccinia	Skin inoculation against smallpox		Exudate	Infected calf lymph i.e. smallpox vaccine	Ward except in cases of severe generalized rash
Adenovirus group					
31 serological types	Inhalation Contact	Pharyngitis Conjunctivitis	Respiratory secretions Conjunctival secretions	Cases Contact, eye instruments	Avoid overcrowding
	Ingestion	Mesenteric adenitis Latent infection in lymphoid tissue, e.g. tonsils and adenoids	Faeces		
Herpes group					
Herpes simplex I	Contact	**Primary** Usually early in life (*a*) symptomless (*b*) gingivostomatitis (*c*) conjunctivitis	Secretions and exudates	Cases	Avoid contact with infants and patients with eczema
	Inoculation	Whitlow			
Herpes simplex II	Contact	Herpes genitalis	Venereal transmission		
Herpes simplex I and II	CNS via nerve tissue	Encephalitis			

		Recurrent Cold sores Keratoconjunctivitis		Usually autogenous	
Varicella zoster	Inhalation	Primary chickenpox	Saliva. Skin lesions	Cases	Isolate for 7 days from rash appearing
	Virus latent in nerve	Recurrent shingles		Autogenous	Segregate from non-immune to varicella
Cytomegalovirus	Blood stream	**Neonatal** generalized infection	Saliva Urine	In utero from mother	
		Children—Hepatitis **Adult**— (*a*) Inapparent glandular fever type (*b*) General infection in lowered resistance, e.g. immunosuppression		Opportunist organism, most adults are symptomless, latent carriers	
Infectious mononucleosis	Mouth	Glandular fever	Throat secretions	Probably close contact with case or carrier, e.g. kissing	Avoid close contact
Epstein-Barr (EB)		Associated with Burkitt's lymphoma			
Myxovirus group					
Influenza A Influenza B	Inhalation	Epidemic influenza Outbreaks of influenza	Droplets of saliva	Cases	Single room until temperature normal for 48 hours
Influenza C		Very occasionally pathogenic			

Virus	*Entry Route*	*Disease*	*Exit Route*	*Usual Sources of Infection*	*Accommodation*
Paramyxovirus group					
Parainfluenza I, II, III, IV	Inhalation	Croup (<5 years)	Droplet infection	Cases	Segregate from babies
Respiratory syncytial virus	Inhalation	Bronchiolitis (<5 years) usually <1 year	Droplet infection	Cases	Segregate from babies
Mumps	Mouth	Mumps	Saliva		Single room for 7 days
Measles	Inhalation	Measles	Droplet infection		Single room until rash fades + 2 days
Rubella	Inhalation	German measles	Droplet infection	Cases and congenital cases	Avoid contact with susceptible women in early pregnancy
Virus hepatitis					
Virus A	Ingestion	Infectious hepatitis	Faeces, urine	Close contact with cases Contaminated water, food and sometimes shellfish	Preferably single room
Virus B	Parenteral inoculation Probably sometimes by injection	Serum hepatitis	Blood. Possibly other bodily excretions and secretions	Contact with infected blood via needles, blood transfusion, communal syringes, tattooing, etc. Probably sexual partners	Preferably single room
Coronavirus group	Inhalation	Respiratory disease	Droplet infection	Cases	

Picornavirus group					
Rhinoviruses 50 serotypes	Inhalation	Common colds	Respiratory secretions	Cases	Single room during acute phase (assisted respiration may be required if respiratory muscles are involved in poliomyelitis)
Enteroviruses (*a*) Poliovirus (*b*) Echovirus (*c*) Coxsackie virus A	Ingestion Multiply in the alimentary tract Spread from gut to tissues, CNS or organs via the blood stream	Often symptomless Poliomyelitis Aseptic meningitis Hand, foot, and mouth disease Herpangina	Faeces Pharyngeal secretions	Cases Poor hygiene and living conditions Symptom free carriers	
Coxsackie virus B		Aseptic meningitis Bornholm disease Myocarditis, pericarditis Aseptic meningitis			
Reovirus group					
Rotavirus	Ingestion	Gastroenteritis < 3 years	Faeces	Contaminated food/milk	Segregate from < 3 years
Arbovirus group					
About 50 serotypes cause disease in man	Inoculation	Yellow fever Systemic febrile disease Encephalitis (not G.B.)	Blood	Birds and mammals via bite of mosquito,tick or sandfly	Mosquito nets
Arenovirus group					
Lassa fever virus	Probably ingestion/ inhalation	Lassa fever	Blood Urine Pharyngeal secretions	Food and environment contaminated by tropical rat urine/saliva Cases	Designated isolation unit
Rhabdovirus group	Inoculation Spread to CNS via nerves	Rabies (fatal acute disease of CNS)	Saliva Urine	Dogs, cats, bats, carnivorous wild animals (G.B. free from rabies due to quarantine)	Isolation unit for duration of illness

Virus	*Entry Route*	*Disease*	*Exit Route*	*Usual Source of Infection*	*Accommodation*
Papovavirus group					
Wart virus	Inoculation	Common warts Venereal warts	Material from wart	Cases	
Rickettsiae					
R. prowazeki	Inoculation (often from infected louse faeces by scratching)	Epidemic typhus fever	Infection of another louse which bites the patient	Alimentary tract of infected lice	
R. tsutsugamushi	Inoculation by bite	Scrub typhus		Infected mites Reservoir, small mammals	
R. burneti	Inhalation Ingestion	Q fever (PUO, atypical pneumonia, endocarditis)		Infected animal faeces Infected cows' milk Placenta, fetal fluids and membranes	
R. mooseri	Inoculation	Endemic typhus fever		Rat fleas	
Chlamydiae	Inhalation	Psittacosis (ornithosis)	Respiratory secretions	Parrots, budgerigars and many birds	Single room during acute febrile phase
	Inoculation by contact	Lymphogranuloma venereum	Discharge from lesions	Cases. Venereal contact	
	Contact	TRIC virus (trachoma, inclusion conjunctivitis) Keratoconjunctivitis and related conditions	Discharge from lesions	Associated with overcrowding and poor sanitation in tropical countries. Fomites, flies	Single room for 48 hours tetracycline or sulphonamide then ward
		Non-specific urethritis and cervicitis	Discharge from lesions	Venereal transmission	

11 Applied Microbiology

To prevent the transmission of infection it is necessary to understand how and why it occurs. Information contained in the preceding chapters must now be applied to hospital nursing practice. It is proposed to do this by the application of general principles which apply to all hospital departments rather than dealing with each department separately, in detail.

Hospitals vary considerably in size, location and age. They have in common a difference from any other buildings: they all provide accommodation for a concentration of sick people of whom a high proportion are at risk from infection because of an injury, surgery, or a disease which destroys the natural protective physiological barriers, and amongst these patients are others admitted for treatment of an existing infection. A well designed, air conditioned modern hospital may be virtually sterile before occupation; add people, and inevitably pathogenic organisms are added at the same time. All staff and patients carry organisms, some are also healthy carriers of pathogenic bacteria, others are known to be infected. Unless operational policies and procedure techniques are related to knowledge of the behaviour of micro-organisms (i.e. the conditions and situations in which growth and multiplication occur, and the mechanisms of transmission) the hospital acquired infection rate may well be higher in a new unit than in a well disciplined old one. New buildings are not the solution to all problems of infection and its control.

Conditions Predisposing to Infection

Bacteria are commonly found in many parts of the body (Chapter 4). The tissue hosts and the parasitic organisms are, as it were, perfectly matched as long as the tissues are healthy, but this equilibrium may easily be upset. Trauma of tissue, as a result of diet or some other irritant, poor aeration of the lungs due to faulty posture, perhaps in bed, debility of tissue due to faulty circulation of blood or inadequate nutrition may reduce the natural resistance of the host and give the organism opportunity for rapid development; hence the boil, the hypostatic pneumonia, the bedsore. Understanding of cause and effect can lead to the prevention of many of these complications. These are examples of endogenous infection, not cross infection, but this is an important aspect of protective patient care.

Bacteria will always multiply rapidly in waste matter which is present where conditions are favourable to organic growth, that is where there is moisture and warmth. Hence a haematoma under a surgical wound, residual urine in a partially obstructed or partially emptied bladder, excess fluid in a joint, are all especially liable to infection. It is, of course, equally true that gross trauma of surface structures as in burns, scalds or crush wounds, by the destruction of tissue which occurs, also provides the ideal situation in which bacteria can flourish, and the most scrupulous asepsis must be observed.

Where tissues offer poor natural resistance to infection, the risk of infection is greatly increased and invasion by a very small number of organisms will cause severe disease, e.g. the inside of the eye and the meninges. In such cases inadequate skin preparation, faulty sterilization of instruments or a lapse in aseptic technique may result in very serious infection.

In certain conditions, e.g. agranulocytosis, hypogammaglobulinaemia, or accidental over-exposure to ionizing radiation, the normal immune mechanisms of the body (Chapter 5) may be impaired or destroyed. In the treatment of other diseases, e.g. certain malignant tumours, leukaemia, or in an attempt to prevent the rejection of a transplanted organ, a similar state is induced by the administration of corticosteroids, cytotoxic, anti-metabolic or immunosuppressive drugs. These patients are at particularly high risk from infection and like patients with extensive burns require a very high standard of nursing and medical care in a protective environment (p. 191).

TRANSMISSION OF INFECTION

Endogenous infection is literally 'from within', i.e. the causative organism comes from another part of the victim's own body.

Exogenous infection is infection originating outside the body, i.e. acquired from another person or object, cross infection.

Endogenous Transfer

A patient or his attendants may inadvertently or carelessly transfer commensal organisms from their normal sites where they are harmless, to another site in the body such as a wound, a pressure sore or tracheostomy, or to equipment such as urine drainage or intravenous infusion apparatus where they can cause infection. For example every patient carries *E. coli* and *Proteus* spp. in the faeces; these easily pass through toilet paper to contaminate the hands; if the hands are not washed the bacteria may be transferred to a vulnerable site to cause infection. During bowel surgery, intestinal organisms may be transferred to the abdominal wall and incision line and cause postoperative wound infection; this is the reason for the meticulous theatre procedure of keeping instruments, swabs and gloves used in contact with the opened bowel separate from those used for the remainder of the operation.

Other commensals are transferred or cause infection only when the surrounding tissue is damaged. For example, *Streptococcus viridans* is always present in the mouth but it can produce dental infection and is forced into the blood stream when a tooth is extracted. If the patient also has diseased heart valves this organism may colonize them and cause subacute bacterial endocarditis.

Symptom-free carriers of pathogenic organisms may

disseminate them to other areas where they will cause infection. For example a throat carrier of *Streptococcus pyogenes* (β-haemolytic *Streptococcus* Group A) may develop a septic finger from the same germ if she sucks her grazed or burnt finger to relieve the pain. Many patients, and up to 50% of hospital staff are nasal carriers of *Staphylococcus aureus,* the organism which causes boils and sepsis.

From the nose, staphylococci are easily transferred to handerkerchiefs, pockets, facecloths, towels, bedding and clothes but particularly to hands, and from any of these contacts to wounds or abrasions to cause infection. Shaving, however skilfully executed, abrades the skin often visibly. If preoperative shaving is scheduled too early, the staphylococci have an opportunity to invade and multiply rapidly in the damaged skin and will be present in very large numbers by the time the patient goes to the operating theatre. The risk of wound infection occurring after incision through such an area is obvious.

Transmission of Infection—Cross Infection

There are four factors essential to the transmission of infection from one person to another:

1. An organism capable of invading and causing infection (Chapter 9).
2. An environment favourable to the growth of that organism (Chapter 4).
3. A transfer mechanism.
4. A susceptible host (Chapter 4).

Organisms capable of causing infection, a favourable environment, and susceptible hosts always exist in a hospital; they can be reduced or separated but not necessarily eliminated. Control of infection measures are therefore often directed towards preventing the essential linking factor from becoming established, i.e. in recognizing and controlling transfer mechanisms, whether human, animal or inanimate. This is the principle underlying operating theatre procedures and aseptic techniques as well as barrier nursing procedures.

The provision of safely sterilized equipment, clean food, well ventilated and clean clinical areas and safe disposal methods are of critical importance but will be ineffective in preventing infection unless allied with the disciplines of hand washing, aseptic technique, and the personal factors such as clean uniform, the proper use of protective clothing, short clean finger nails, hair styled so that it does not swing and disseminate bacteria (or become contaminated) and a conscientious attitude towards minor infections such as styes, boils and sore throats.

Hospital Environmental Factors

New hospitals are being built, experienced nurses are working with planning teams and many more nurses are consulted about the detail of ward and departmental plans. From the infection control viewpoint several factors should be mentioned:

1. The design should facilitate good practice, e.g. clear definition of clean and dirty areas, an adequate number of wash hand basins in appropriate places.

2. In a general hospital at least 25% of the beds should be in *single rooms* with facilities for hand washing and storage for protective clothing in *anterooms* so that infected patients and those at risk from infection can be effectively segregated and safely nursed.

3. *Beds* should be spaced to allow correct working procedures and so that respiratory organisms are not directly transmitted from one patient to the next. As a working guide, bed centres should be at least 2·5 m apart and where beds are opposite to each other a distance of not less than 2 m between foot ends is recommended (Department of Health and Social Security 1968). Overcrowding increases the risk of cross infection.

4. Careful *selection of surfaces* and finishes is necessary so that they are not only aesthetically pleasing but can be efficiently and economically cleaned. The

modern trend towards carpeting even clinical areas has been shown by some careful scientific studies to have microbiological dangers in the accumulation of bacteria within the pile, as well as the obvious difficulty of removing hospital spills, blood, urine or chemicals. Basin and bath overflow drains should be omitted, they are impossible to keep clean and are commonly heavily contaminated with *Pseudomonas aeruginosa* and coliform organisms which may be splashed back on to the hands during washing.

5. The provision of *adequate ventilation* in a hospital is not as simple as it would at first appear. Stairwells, lifts and chutes as well as doors and windows have an effect on the movement and direction of air flow in a multi-storey building. Opening the windows in a ward to produce a current of fresh air not only makes the atmosphere more pleasant, it also reduces the number of organisms by diluting the concentration present. In the operating theatre where tissues normally protected by the skin and other natural barriers, are exposed for a considerable time it is important for the air to be as clean as possible; air is therefore filtered, humidified, warmed or cooled, delivered and extracted at a measured rate by the air conditioning plant. The circulation and direction in which air flows is also important; theatre suites are described in zones, 'sterile', clean, dirty, the pressure being highest in the sterile preparation room and theatre, and lowest in the changing and sluice rooms so that the air flows from sterile to clean to dirty zones, never in reverse.

In patient protection units as well as in operating theatres the aims are:

a. To introduce pathogen-free air.
b. To prevent contaminated air entering by other routes, e.g. doors.
c. To minimize contamination from the environment.
d. To remove bacteria as rapidly as possible from the vicinity of the patient.

The median diameter of pathogenic bacteria-carrying particles in air is about 12 μm, range 4–24. In practice filters with 99·9% efficiency at 5 μm pass air suitable for operating theatre suites (p. 84).

Laminar air flow clean rooms have recently received publicity for their use in hospital in operating theatres, organ transplant and special care units. In a laminar air flow room, air moving at high speed (often 30 m per minute) is introduced through a filter bank which takes the place of the whole of one wall (horizontal flow) or the entire ceiling (vertical flow) and is extracted through the opposite wall in the first case and at floor level in the other. The principal advantage of laminar air flow ventilation is the rate at which the organisms are removed from the vicinity of the patient. Provided that neither person nor object moves or projects between the air source (i.e. one wall in horizontal flow or the ceiling in vertical flow) and the patient the possibility of transfer of organisms is minimal. This fact in no way diminishes the possibility of contact transmission by staff carrying out medical or nursing procedures, or of self contamination by the patient.

6. Animals and insects can spread disease. Hospitals, particularly the kitchens, should be designed to exclude this possibility, e.g. fly screens, rat proof stores.

Clean and Sterile Supplies

Food. Contaminated food, milk, water or ice may cause outbreaks of food poisoning, e.g. due to staphylococcal enterotoxin, *Clostridium welchii, Salmonella* or *Shigella,* or a disease such as typhoid fever, tuberculosis or brucellosis. The staff and all patients are susceptible, babies under a year old are at particularly high risk because they lack one of the natural defence barriers to intestinal infection, stomach hydrochloric acid.

Patients receiving extensive antibiotic therapy, those with low white blood cell counts and babies are also very susceptible to mouth infection caused by *Candida* sp. (*Monilia,* thrush) which is easily spread from patient to patient by inadequately processed feeding equipment and crockery, e.g. cups, bottle teats, medicine spoons and glasses. Other organisms such as *Streptococcus pyogenes* or tubercle bacilli may be transferred in this way, the bacteria being protected in inaccessible cracks or in dried sputum or saliva. There is no place for perfunctory washing-up procedures or the use of cracked or chipped crockery. If a washing-up machine with liberal supplies of very hot water is not available, it is necessary to boil utensils after their use by a patient with any mouth or throat infection.

In this country there are statutory regulations concerning food supplies. Certain standards are required in restaurants and institutions; these relate to kitchen hygiene, the storage and handling of food, staff health, conditions of work and personal hygiene, e.g. the provision of clean uniform, hand-washing and toilet facilities. Staff with diarrhoea and vomiting, septic lesions, or respiratory tract infections must be excluded from duty. Prevention of infection transmitted in food is also dependent on scrupulous cleanliness in the ward kitchens, paediatric feed kitchens, ice making machines, and any containers or conveyors used for transporting food. It is not always appreciated that ice is very readily contaminated, often with coliform organisms (p. 75) and that cold inhibits but does not destroy bacteria. Ward kitchen refrigerators should be reserved for food storage and require regular cleaning. Drugs, blood and clinical specimens awaiting transport to the laboratory should be kept in a separate refrigerator.

Thorough hand-washing to remove transient contaminating bacteria is essential before preparing or serving food or feeding a patient. An additional, but wise precaution is to exclude from the ward kitchen, all patients, staff handling bedpans of patients suspected or known to have *Salmonella* or *Shigella* infection, and staff changing napkins of any baby with intestinal symptoms.

Sterile supplies. Sterile supplies used in a hospital come from various sources; they may be commercially prepacked and sterilized, supplied by a local or regional

Central Sterile Supply Department (CSSD), by the pharmacy, or processed in a department such as an operating theatre. While it is usually the responsibility of the bacteriologist and the Control of Infection Committee to advise on methods of sterilization, packaging, and safe storage and the responsibility of the Nursing Procedure Committee to advise on selection, opening and procedure, it is the responsibility of every user to check that each pack is undamaged before use and opened in the prescribed manner so that the sterility of the content is preserved.

Sterilizing methods are discussed in Chapter 7 and *indicators* in Appendix I. The outer container should be labelled with the method and date of processing, and an appropriate sterilizing indicator. The *packing and presentation of sterile supplies* is subject to central as well as local control. Many pharmaceutical preparations are manufactured to exacting requirements; expert committees convened by the Department of Health and Social Security study and recommend standards for packaging materials and methods of packing; the Steering Committee on Standardization of Supplies from CSSD which includes nurse members, has produced an interim report (1970) on the content and presentation of certain ward and obstetric packs.

Packaging materials should facilitate sterilization, for example, allow steam penetration, but also act as a barrier to insects, dust or moisture which could carry bacteria into the pack. Incorrect packing or wrapping will invalidate the sterilizing procedure. For example, nylon film is steam permeable but the time taken to evacuate air from the pack and achieve steam penetration is far in excess of the normal autoclave cycle time, making this an unsuitable wrap for this sterilization method. Substandard paper bags or inadequately heat-sealed plastic or paper, or poor fold closures will allow pack content contamination after sterilization.

In considering the *storage of sterile supplies* the aim is to preserve sterility not to challenge it with severe tests. It is therefore recommended that:

1. Supplies are stored well off the floor, in a clean, dry area.

2. In an even temperature.

3. Protected from dust. Any accumulated dust will be disseminated at the time of opening and is likely to settle on the sterile field.

4. Shelf and container surfaces should be smooth for ease of cleaning and to prevent damage to the packs.

5. Supplies should be used in strict rotation to avoid deterioration.

6. 'Shelf life' (prescribed storage time) will depend to some extent on local conditions. It is generally agreed that paper-wrapped packs present the problem. Waterproof plastic and metal can be swabbed with a suitable antiseptic to remove accumulated dust, which in a hospital is likely to contain pathogens. Given intact and efficient wraps, it is probable that sterilized pack contents remain sterile for a long time but in the case of paper-wrapped packs (where damp swabbing to remove dust would certainly contaminate the content) it is impossible to open the pack without contaminating the content with the dust which has collected on the outer wrap. Double wraps are considered to be safer than a single layer because the inner wrap acts as a barrier to dust and bacteria disturbed when the outer layer is opened. The longer a pack is stored, the more dust accumulates on the outside, and the greater the chance of contamination on opening. For this reason turnover should be as fast as possible to ensure the shortest practicable shelf life.

Many pharmaceutical preparations are marked with an expiry date after which they should not be used, others have a colour indicator incorporated which changes when the chemical loses its activity.

It is easy and wrong to assume that all lotions, ointments, creams and antiseptics in the ward cupboards are sterile. Fluids, including antiseptics, are very easily contaminated by contact with a hand, a swab or a dropped and replaced stopper. An antiseptic may be effective against one group of bacteria but totally ineffective against another group, e.g. cetrimide is active against staphylococci but will allow *Pseudomonas aeruginosa* to survive; staphylococci unlike most other organisms can survive in saline. A Winchester of distilled water used to 'top-up' humidifiers, although sterile when issued, may easily become contaminated by a wet medium organism such as *Klebsiella* sp. which will then multiply, infect the humidifier at the next filling, and then the patient. Hand cream by the ward basin, contaminated by an unwashed hand may pass a pathogenic organism on to the next user who washes before carrying out a clean procedure for a patient. Patients should be supplied with individual containers of creams or ointments, particularly when they are to be applied to the skin by hand. Recommendations in 1969 (HM(69)86 *Preservation of sterility in ophthalmic preparations used in hospitals),* concerning eye medications emphasize the serious risk of cross infection where communal stock containers of eye drops or ointments are used. Each patient should have his own drops or ointments applied with a sterilized pipette or rod, or single dose applicators should be used.

Clean supplies. A critical appraisal of items of equipment which are either communal or used by a succession of patients will underline the necessity for thorough cleaning and effective decontamination between patients to prevent the spread of infection by indirect contact. For example:

Mouth and respiratory tract infections, e.g. *Streptococcus pyogenes* or *Candida* sp., may be transmitted by nursing equipment such as thermometers, inhalation or oral hygiene equipment as well as by incubators, respirators and humidifiers.

Staphylococcus aureus is easily transferred from skin to talcum powder used for pressure area care, and thence to every patient in the ward if a communal tin is used. A culture of the 'tide line' of a bath or washing bowl grows skin and intestinal organisms, an obvious hazard to another user with an imperfectly healed wound.

Communal towels, wheel chair blankets, bath mats, soft toys or pillows not enclosed in plastic cases show bacteriological evidence of all their recent users and may be responsible for an outbreak of cross infection.

Communal items are always bacteriologically suspect.

Aseptic Technique

An eminent surgeon performing a difficult operation, a radiographer or physiotherapist replacing a dressing, a physician aspirating a chest, a medical student or house officer passing a catheter, an anaesthetist giving a spinal anaesthetic, and a nurse removing stitches or aspirating a tracheostomy all practice aseptic technique based on the same principles, and with the same aim: to carry out a procedure without introducing micro-organisms directly or indirectly to the vulnerable tissues of the patient.

PRINCIPLES AND REQUIREMENTS

1. A **clean environment** and adequate working space.

2. Sterile dressings, instruments, lotions and equipment (Chapter 7).

3. **Skin preparation.** Skin and hair are never sterile. In addition to the normal skin flora (p. 23) both pick up and transiently carry any organisms with which they are in contact. This is one reason (see also p. 176) for the preoperative shaving of patient's body hair, and for covering the hair of staff working in operating theatres and other high risk areas. Both the skin of the patient and the hands of the operator are thoroughly washed and dried to remove transient contaminating bacteria, particular attention being paid to skin creases, e.g. between the fingers, the umbilicus, etc. To remove any remaining surface bacteria an antiseptic, e.g. iodine, chlorhexidine, is applied to the operation area before the skin is incised or punctured.

4. Prevent organisms from the operator from reaching vulnerable patient tissues, by the use of **protective clothing** and **non-touch technique**.

Caps. Hair should always be restrained since it disperses bacteria freely when moving. It should be completely covered by a cap when this constitutes a risk to the patient, e.g. for protective (reverse) barrier nursing, in the operating theatre or the intensive therapy unit.

Masks. Masks are made from various materials, e.g. paper, plastic foam, cotton fabric with a cellophane insert, glass fibre. They function either by deflecting expired air, e.g. simple paper type, or by filtration, e.g. close fitting glass fibre type. Respiratory organisms in deflected air will land in the room but away from the immediate area; they will be trapped in the fibres of the filtration type of mask. Both types of mask are effective only when dry.

Many hospitals do not use masks for minor procedures, where this is the policy it should be remembered that while quiet breathing disseminates very few bacteria from the nose and throat; talking, laughing, coughing and sneezing disseminate very large numbers. Where masks are worn they should be discarded when not required; handling a used mask, storing it in a pocket or wearing it intermittently dropped around the neck are serious infection risks.

Gloves. To avoid direct contact between the skin of the operator and the patient either non-touch technique, i.e. the use of forceps instead of fingers, is used or sterile gloves are worn. Dressings and sterile equipment are handled by the same means to avoid indirect transmission of organisms.

Gowns. Skin particles and bacteria are constantly shed, the clothing and shoes of a normal individual carry these and other micro-organisms picked up by contact with people and objects. The clothing of hospital staff moving from patient to patient may be very heavily contaminated and for this reason a clean gown (sterile in certain situations) is worn when carrying out aseptic procedures.

Closely woven fabric is a barrier to bacteria when dry

but allows them to pass in both directions when wet. If a surgeon gets his sterile gown wet with blood or saline, bacteria from the patient will be in contact with his skin, conversely bacteria from the surgeon's skin and the clothing under his gown will gain access to the wound. It is most important for all members of the staff to change into freshly laundered theatre clothing and theatre shoes before entering the clean zone of the operating theatre or other area where patients are at high risk from infection and every effort is made to keep the numbers of micro-organisms to the minimum.

5. **Clean procedures** should always be carried out before those known or suspected to be infected.

6. When **opening ward procedure packs:** (*a*) Check that the pack is undamaged. (*b*) Check that the pack has been through a sterilizing process (indicator). (*c*) Check that the prescribed storage time has not been exceeded. (*d*) Tearing paper disperses fragments and dust from the surface, therefore the *outer bag* of packs other than those designed to peel open or to unfold, should be cut with clean scissors reserved for this purpose. (*e*) The *inner wrapper* of the pack is opened to form the sterile field by handling the corners of the wrapper only, opening away from the body first so that it is never necessary to reach across the *sterile field*. (*f*) Only sterile materials are placed on the sterile field, these and the field itself are only touched by sterile forceps or by sterile gloved hands. Once sterile swabs have been in contact with the patient's wound and skin they are no longer sterile, therefore they are never replaced on the sterile field or redipped into sterile lotion but discarded and a new swab taken.

7. **Safe disposal** of all used material is an important aspect of infection control. Used dressings and instruments should be contained at the point of use, in suitable waterproof bags for transportation to the incinerator and service departments.

'REVERSE' BARRIER: HIGH DEGREE PROTECTION FROM INFECTION

Certain patients are at very high risk from infection, including infections which would be trivial to a healthy person. Some, for instance patients with extensive skin destruction or burns, have lost a first-line defence mechanism to invasion by bacteria. Others have compromised immune responses (Chapter 5). This group includes patients with agranulocytosis, accidentally drug-induced or due to primary disease, and those who are receiving immunosuppressive therapy. In addition to the nursing care required for such a clinical condition, these patients need a degree of protection from infection comparable with that found in a well organized operating theatre. That is, a scrupulously clean environment, everything coming into contact with the patient sterilized or as free from micro-organisms as its construction will allow, and a team which is well disciplined in aseptic technique including the use of protective clothing.

The aim is to protect the patient from contact with organisms from other people, directly by skin contact or from the respiratory tract, or indirectly via food, drugs, medical and nursing equipment, all of which have to be sterilized.

The greatest risk to the patient comes from other people. Objects can be rendered free from micro-organisms, people cannot. For this reason these patients are ideally nursed in specially designed isolators or units which provide a controlled environment and restrict access. Some isolators of the 'plastic bubble' type are designed to allow the staff to give patient care through sterile gloves or a half-suit, set in the side wall of the 'bubble', thus preventing direct human contact. No one other than the patient ever enters the unit. In other special units the minimum number of staff, wearing full protective clothing, enter to give care or treatment. It is most important for these people to have a responsible attitude to minor infections which could have serious consequences if transmitted to the patient.

It is possible to adapt a single room with good nursing facilities to give a reasonable degree of protection provided that access is strictly limited and anything taken into the room is sterilized or as free from organisms as possible.

PRINCIPLES OF NURSING CARE OF INFECTED PATIENTS

Isolation nursing implies segregation of staff, patients and accommodation; it can therefore only be carried out where separate wards and staff facilities are available. Patients known to have specific infectious fevers, e.g. measles or smallpox, those with transmissible diseases, e.g. open pulmonary tuberculosis, and sometimes those with very severe drug-resistant infection are transferred to such units.

Barrier nursing is the discipline necessary for the safe nursing care of patients with existing or hospital acquired infection, in multi-bedded wards and their associated single side wards which also house uninfected patients. The aim is to prevent the transmission of pathogenic micro-organisms directly, or indirectly via air-borne particles, fluids, equipment or food, to other patients, staff or visitors. Many hospitals have only a limited number of single rooms which have to be allocated to the best advantage of all patients; from the infection control viewpoint it is necessary to segregate infected patients who are a danger to others, and patients who are at very high risk from infection. It is not easy to achieve efficient barrier nursing practice other than in a single room with an ante-room with protective clothing and hand washing facilities, but the risks of transmitting bacteria can always be greatly reduced by identifying the causative organism, the sites and media in which it flourishes, the methods of spread, and applying this knowledge to institute appropriate barriers. The following should always be checked:

1. What is the causative organism?
2. Where is it?
3. By which route does it leave the body?
4. Are other patients or staff in the ward vulnerable?
5. Is segregation essential, advisable, or unnecessary?

General Principles

1. The environment is kept clean and well ventilated to reduce the numbers of organisms.

2. Unwashed hands of staff moving from one patient or his equipment to another are the most common agents of infection transmission. Always wash and dry hands after contact with an infected patient or his personal effects and bedding.

3. Bacteria are able to pass freely, rapidly, and in both directions through *moist media* including saturated wound dressings and drainage equipment.

4. Limit the number of people in direct contact with an infected patient, e.g. by restricting contact with other patients and visitors if necessary, by selecting a suitably sited bed, by allocating one nurse only on each shift to carry out infected patient care.

5. Check the immunization status of the staff so that they are not exposed to unnecessary risk, e.g. in tuberculosis, diphtheria, poliomyelitis.

6. Infected material is safely contained at the point of use and subsequently destroyed or decontaminated. Polythene or wet strength paper bags of different colours to distinguish combustible, non-combustible waste, and items for decontamination and reprocessing, e.g. linen, are safe, take up little space and can be securely closed.

The use of 'disposables', e.g. protective clothing, bed 'linen', eating utensils, as well as medical and nursing equipment has obvious advantages provided that storage space and an efficient means of destruction are available.

Excreta and secretions should be disposed directly into the main sewage system, i.e. water closet or bedpan washer. In certain circumstances, for example areas without or with inadequate methods of sewage disposal, it may be necessary to disinfect excreta by thoroughly mixing it with a suitable disinfectant, e.g. hypochlorite in poliomyelitis, phenol/cresol in enteric infection, in the bedpan. Cover to exclude flies during the holding time before disposal.

Crockery and cutlery must be free from cracks and chips. They can be safely processed in an efficiently functioning washing up machine; failing this, they should be washed under running water and then boiled. The practice of keeping marked crockery in the ward kitchen or patient's room is unsatisfactory.

Mattresses and pillows should be sealed into impervious covers, e.g. polythene which can be discarded, or processed in a high vacuum autoclave before use by another patient. Low temperature steam with formaldehyde is also used to disinfect bedding. In the absence of modern laundry facilities which include safe handling methods, pre-wash sluicing and high temperature washing cycles, infected linen should be totally immersed and soaked in a suitable disinfectant solution, e.g. phenol/cresol, before laundering.

Comparative Notes on Barrier Nursing in a Single Bed Sideward

	To Segregate for Infection	*To Segregate for Patient Protection*
Aim	The patient has an infection Anything coming out of the room must be disinfected or safely contained for disposal	The patient is particularly vulnerable, requires protection from infection. Anything going into the room should be free from organisms capable of causing infection
Visitors	Exclude other patients Instruct family	Essential staff and selected visitors only, to reduce the risk of contact transmission
Door	Closed Label 'Barrier Nursing'	Closed. Label 'Barrier Nursing For Patient Protection'
Hand washing	On leaving (and for procedures)	On entering (and for procedures)
Gown	To protect staff clothing Store clean supply outside room Discard inside room, contain in polythene bag	To protect the patient from staff clothing. Store clean supply outside room Discard outside room
Mask	Only if spread of infection is by airborne droplets. Worn to prevent a large dose of bacteria being directly inhaled Discard inside room	Always Efficient filtration type Put on before entry Discard outside room
Cap		Completely cover the hair
Gloves	For serum hepatitis if handling blood, secretions or excreta For intestinal infections when the patient is incontinent	Sterile gloves for aseptic procedures, e.g. intravenous infusion
Crockery etc.	Disposable Efficiently functioning washing up machine Wash and boil Condiments, sugar, kept in room	Process utensils through the washing up machine immediately before serving meal
Food	Normal Incinerate any waste	Serve before other patients Select foods which have not been handled after cooking AVOID trifles, salads, milk from open jugs, etc
Amenities	Paperback books. Incinerate. Toys etc. should be disposable or of material which can be sterilized after use	Avoid items which have been used by other patients Newspapers will autoclave! Plants and flower water are frequently colonized by wet medium organisms, e.g. *Pseudomonas aeruginosa*
Furniture and equipment	Minimum Select smooth, intact surfaces for ease of cleaning Freshly laundered, frequently changed, curtains No carpets or mats Individual medicines, lotions and ointments	
Bed and personal linen	Clean daily	

Comparative Notes on Barrier Nursing in a Single Bed Sideward *(contd.)*.

	To Segregate for Infection	*To Segregate for Patient Protection*
Room cleaning	Surfaces	Damp dust with paper towels or disposable cloths Discard in the room disposal bag
	Basin	Clean with paper towels It is most important to keep traps and overflows clean
	Floor	Separate bucket and disposable-head mop, kept in the patient's room or in a separate cupboard Wet clean with detergent and a suitable disinfectant N.B. The disinfectant must be compatible with both the detergent and the plastic material of the mop head
Terminal disinfection	Patient	Bath and move into a clean bed
	Equipment	Collect into designated polythene bags: (*a*) Laundry (*b*) Combustible waste (*c*) Non-combustible waste (*d*) Pillows for autoclaving (*e*) Surgical equipment for return to CSSD or central disinfection
	Room	The room should be thoroughly cleaned, the bed, furniture, fittings and any remaining equipment, e.g. bed cradle, washed with detergent in hot water, dried, and left to air for 24 hours before further use. Cloths used for this purpose are discarded.

Appendix I

Sterilization Indicators and Tests

AUTOCLAVE CONTROL AND TESTING

Engineers Department	Correct installation with service access. Planned maintenance. (Department of Health and Social Security, Hospital Technnical Memorandum No. 10 *Steam Sterilizers.*) Training of the operator.

Autoclave Process Indicators

Temperature and pressure charts record and present a visual check on the autoclave cycle, steam temperatures and pressures.

Thermometers in the outlet drain and the load simulator register accurate temperatures inside the autoclave; these are displayed on dials on the control panel.

Sterilization Process Indicators

These are placed in or on each pack to show that it has been through a satisfactory sterilizing process.

Heat/moisture-sensitive tape is plain before autoclaving and develops dark brown stripes or pattern after exposure to steam at sterilizing time/temperature.

Heat-sensitive dyes and inks. These vary in reliability. Colour change.

Heat-sensitive chemicals, e.g. Browne's sterilizer control tubes which contain a chemical which reacts to heat, turning slowly from red (unsterile) to yellow to green. Green indicates satisfactory time/temperature exposure.

Thermolabile plastic melts at a given temperature and flows to a mark on the enclosing tube or sachet. Failure to reach the mark indicates sterilization failure.

Autoclave Tests

Thermocouple. This is a temperature recording instrument used to monitor load conditions. One or more sensors (fine probes consisting of two different metals, e.g. copper/constantan) are positioned at test points within the autoclave load, the leads are channelled out through valves in the autoclave wall and linked to a galvanometer, the dial of which gives a constant reading of the temperatures at the test points.

Bowie-Dick test. This is a test to detect any air remaining or leaking into a high vacuum autoclave during the cycle. Procedure see Fig. 47. It is not a suitable test for any other type of autoclave.

Air leak test. This is a method of detecting air leaking into the chamber through a faulty valve or door seal. The autoclave is closed, the vacuum drawn on manual control, and the valves then closed to isolate the chamber. The vacuum should be maintained; a decrease in vacuum of more than 10 mmHg during 10 minutes holding time indicates an air leak and the machine requires servicing by an engineer before use. Test for high vacuum autoclaves only.

Biological testing. Heat resistant spores, usually of *Bacillus stearothermophilus,* are placed in test packs in a normal load, they are then sent to the laboratory for culture which takes up to five days. Only an efficient

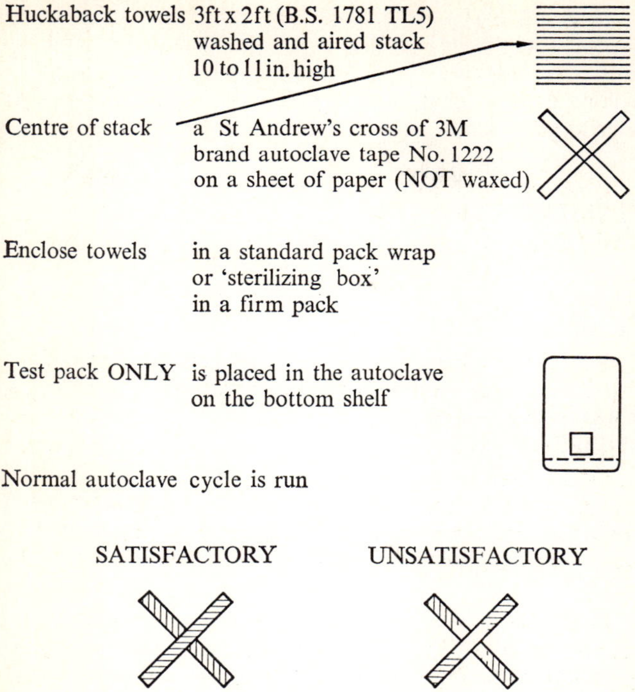

Fig. 47. *The Bowie-Dick autoclave test.*

autoclave will kill these spores. This method of testing is infrequently used for routine purposes, largely because of the time factor.

HOT AIR OVEN TESTS AND INDICATORS

Temperature charts record the time cycle and the temperature within the oven, but not within the load.

Thermocouple testing is essential in order to set the correct time cycle.

Heat-sensitive chemicals or tape are used to indicate by colour change that an item has been through a dry heat sterilizing process. Foil sealing caps often carrying a colour change indicator, a wide range is available, e.g. blue to pink, red to gold.

GAMMA IRRADIATION STERILIZATION INDICATOR

The most commonly used indicator is a small, circular, adhesive disc which changes in colour from yellow to red.

ETHYLENE OXIDE STERILIZATION INDICATOR

Green gas-sensitive tape turns from deep to pale green after exposure to ethylene oxide gas. Care must be taken not to leave an unsterile load in the sterilizer as even traces of the gas will complete the colour change in about 24 hours.

A chemical solution enclosed in a sachet turns from yellow to purple after exposure to ethylene oxide gas. The time taken to effect the change depends on the temperature.

Biological testing. *Bacillus subtilis (globigii)* spores are used.

Appendix II

Environmental Sampling Methods

Fluids	Collect with a sterile syringe and needle. Transfer into a sterile laboratory container.
Surfaces	Use a sterile swab, e.g. throat swab. Moisten with sterile broth or sterile distilled water for dry surfaces. Rotate the swab whilst rubbing it lightly and evenly over the surface.
Fabrics	(*a*) Contact plates. Fabric is pressed lightly on to the surface of an agar plate. Avoid contamination from hands by wearing a disposable polythene glove or 'bunching up' the fabric. (*b*) Sweep plates. An area of fabric 30–60 cm is stretched and an inverted agar plate swept up and down it 10 times with the plate edges in contact with the fabric.
Tubing	Bacteriologists often prefer to sample tubing in the laboratory where it can be sectioned. Sterile broth is injected at one end, allowed to flow slowly through the tubing, and is collected into a sterile laboratory container at the other end. Care must be taken to avoid contamination from the outside of the tubing ends.
Air	(*a*) Flow is observed by tracing smoke generated by, e.g. titanium tetrachloride which forms dense white smoke when in contact with atmospheric moisture. (*b*) Volume and direction are measured with a vane anemometer.

(*c*) Humidity is measured with an hygrometer or calculated from wet and dry bulb thermometer readings.

(*d*) Cleanliness is measured by counting bacteria collected by: (*i*) *settle plates*. Agar plates are exposed for a specified time (usually 15 minutes). Bacteria collected on the surface are identified and counted. (*ii*) *Air sampling machines,* e.g. Bourdillon slit sampler which draws air at the rate of 1 ft^3 per minute, through a narrow slit on to the surface of an agar plate 2 mm below. The plate rests on a small turntable which completes its revolution in a fixed time, for example 5 minutes. The slit equals the radius of the plate. Using such equipment, an accurate estimate of the numbers of bacteria in a room can be made.

IN-USE TESTING OF DISINFECTANTS

Kelsey and Maurer (1974) describe a practical method of sampling and assessing the efficiency of disinfectant solutions which are actually in use in a working situation, e.g. in a urinal disinfection tank or a floor scrubbing machine reservoir. 1 ml of disinfectant solution in use is collected with a sterile pipette and added to 9 ml of diluent in a sterile container. The diluent is selected according to the disinfectant and the site of use, and is supplied by the bacteriology laboratory. The container is sent straight back to the laboratory for processing. Two agar plates are inoculated. One is incubated at 37°C for three days, the other at room temperature for seven days. The plates are then examined and the results reported.

If bacteria are grown the disinfectant fails the test, i.e. is failing to kill bacteria in the situation and in the strength at which it is in use.

Chemical disinfection is unreliable and many hospitals therefore have a routine in-use testing programme.

'SEE FOR YOURSELF'

Respiratory Tract Bacteria

1. Cough on to an agar plate held about 10 cm from the mouth.
2. Compare the telephone mouthpiece of a ward and a public telephone (moistened swab).
3. Swab an oxygen or anaesthetic mask immediately after use.
4. Swab the inside of a used toothmug.

Skin Bacteria

1. Swab a bath 'tide line', clean the bath and swab again. Compare the results.
2. A used communal towel contact plate.
3. Dirty, washed but wet, then well dried hands. In each situation make fingerprints on an agar plate by rolling the tip of each finger in turn lightly on the surface of a separate area of the plate (see Chapter 11).
4. Settle plate exposed in a ward during bedmaking, place on the floor by the end of a bed, expose for 15 minutes. Compare with a plate exposed when the ward is quiet.

Intestinal Bacteria, Wet Medium Bacteria

1. Swab under the rim of a bedpan.
2. The next sheet of toilet paper. Contact plate.
3. Sample of flower water.
4. Kitchen sink cloth. Contact plate.
5. Floor cloth or mop. Contact plate.
6. Drain trap. Sample as far down the drain as can be reached with a throat swab.

Multiplication Factors

Multiplication factor	*Prefix*	*Symbol*
1 000 000 000 000 = 10^{12}	tera	T
1 000 000 000 = 10^{9}	giga	G
1 000 000 = 10^{6}	mega	M
1 000 = 10^{3}	kilo	k
100 = 10^{2}	hecto	h
10 = 10^{1}	deca	da
0·1 = 10^{-1}	deci	d
0·01 = 10^{-2}	centi	c
0· 001 = 10^{-3}	milli	m
0· 000 001 = 10^{-6}	micro	μ
0· 000 000 001 = 10^{-9}	nano	n
0· 000 000 000 001 = 10^{-12}	pico	p
0· 000 000 000 000 001 = 10^{-15}	femto	f
0· 000 000 000 000 000 001 = 10^{-18}	atto	a

Equivalents

mμ = nm = nanometre (10^{-9})
μ = μm = micrometre (10^{-6})

Length:

1 foot = 0·305 metres
3 feet = 0·915 metres

Weight:

2·205 pounds = 1000 grams = 1 kilogram

Energy:

1 calorie = 4·2 joules (J)

Capacity:

1 pint = 0·568 litres

Temperature:

Fahrenheit (F) minus 32 multiplied by 5/9 = C
Celsius (C) multiplied by 9/5 plus 32 = F

$<$ = less than
$>$ = greater than

Selected Further Reading

HISTORY BOOKS

Baldry, P. E. (1976) *The Battle against Bacteria. A History of the Development of Antibacterial Drugs for the General Reader,* 2nd ed. London: Cambridge University Press.

Cuny, H. (1965) *Louis Pasteur: The Man and his Theories,* Translated by Patrick Evans. London: Souvenir Press.

Guthrie, Douglas (1949) *Lord Lister. His Life and Doctrine*. Edinburgh: Livingstone.

Ludovici, L. J. (1958) *The World of the Infinitely Small.* London: Dent.

Manson-Bahr, Sir Philip (1962) *Patrick Manson—The Father of Tropical Medicine*. London: Thomas Nelson.

Maurois, A. (1963) *The Life of Alexander Fleming.* Harmondsworth: Penguin.

Parish, H. J. (1968) *Victory with Vaccine.* Edinburgh: Livingstone.

Wilson, J. R. (1963) *Margin of Safety. The Story of Poliomyelitis Vaccine*. London: Collins.

MICROBIOLOGY BOOKS

Frobisher, M. & others (1969) *Microbiology for Nurses,* 11th ed. Philadelphia: Saunders.

Garrod, L. P. & O'Grady, F. (1973) *Antibiotics and Chemotherapy,* 4th ed. Edinburgh: Livingstone.

Gillies, R. R. & Dodds, T. C. (1976) *Bacteriology Illustrated,* 4th ed. Edinburgh: Livingstone.

Halliday, W. J. (1971) *Glossary of Immunological Terms*. London: Butterworths.

Hynes, M. (1968) *Whitby and Hynes's Medical Bacteriology Including Elementary Mycology and Parasitology,* 9th ed. London: Churchill.

Timbury, M. C. (1974) *Notes for Medical Virology,* 5th ed. Edinburgh: Livingstone.

Weir, D. M. (1973) *Immunology for Undergraduates,* 3rd ed. Edinburgh: Livingstone.

Also:

Christie, A. B. (1974) *Infectious Diseases,* 2nd ed. London: Faber & Faber.

Tighe, J. R. (1972) *Pathology,* 3rd ed. London: Baillière Tindall.

Advanced:

Cruickshank, R. (1972/1975) *Medical Microbiology,* Vols I & II, 12th ed. Edinburgh: Livingstone.

Jawetz, E. & others (1976) *Review of Medical Microbiology,* 12th ed. Calif.: Lange.

Rhodes, A. J. & Van Rooyen, C. E. (1962) *Textbook of Virology*. Baltimore: Williams & Wilkins.

Sykes, G. (1975) *Disinfection and Sterilization,* 2nd ed. London: Chapman & Hall.

APPLIED MICROBIOLOGY BOOKS

Berenson, A. S. (1975) *Control of Communicable Diseases in Man,* 12th ed. American Public Health Association.

Gibson, G. L. (1974) *Infections in Hospitals,* 2nd ed. Edinburgh and London: Churchill Livingstone.

Lowbury, E. J. L. & others (1975) *Control of Hospital Infection*. London: Chapman & Hall.

Maurer, I. M. (1974) *Hospital Hygiene*. London: Edward Arnold.

Parry, W. H. (1973) *Communicable Diseases. An Epidemiological Approach,* 2nd ed. London: English Universities Press.

Smillie, W. G. & Kilbourne, E. D. (1963) *Preventive Medicine and Public Health.* London: Macmillan.

REPORTS AND ARTICLES

Thousands of reports and articles, in English and other languages, are published every year. Regular reading of journals such as *The Nursing Times, The Nursing Mirror,* and the *International Nursing Review* will introduce topics of current concern and interest; some other journals and official bodies which regularly publish important original reports and articles on microbiological topics are listed below. All nurses, in particular those concerned with teaching or infection control should have access to these journals:

British Medical Journal
British Hospital Journal and Social Service Review (publishes the proceedings of the Central Sterilizing Club)
Journal of Clinical Pathology
Journal of Hygiene
Journal of Medical Microbiology
Lancet

Department of Health and Social Security, and *The Scottish Home and Health Department*

A list of publications is available from H.M.S.O. Memoranda to National Health Service Hospitals, e.g. HM(69) 'Preservation of sterility in ophthalmic preparations used in hospitals.'

King Edward's Hospital Fund for London

Also have a reference library and advisory Hospital Centre in London.

The Medical Research Council

E.g. Aseptic methods in the operating suite. A report by the sub-committee on aseptic methods in operating theatres of the Committee on Hospital Infection (1968).
Lancet i, 705, 763, 831.

Nuffield Provincial Hospitals Trust

E.g. *Central Sterile Supply. Principles and Practice* (1963) Oxford University Press.

Public Health Laboratory Service

The weekly Communicable Disease Reports include brief epidemiological studies as well as national statistics.

World Health Organization

WHO Chronicle. A monthly record of WHO assisted health activities for the medical and public health professions.

Bulletin of the WHO. Technical articles by physicians and scientists engaged in public health work.

World Health. An illustrated magazine for the general public. Also technical reports and statistics.

Index